COPING

Ruth Fowke

M.B., B.Ch., D.P.M.

HODDER AND STOUGHTON

Printed in Great Britain for Hodder and Stoughton Limited,
St Paul's House, Warwick Lane, London, E.C.4, by
Cox & Wyman Limited, London, Fakenham and Reading

CONTENTS

CONTENTS

1

FACING A CRISIS

Shortly after I took up psychiatry my brother dropped a deliberate, shattering social brick. Meeting friends of the family who enquired after me he replied, tongue in cheek, 'Oh, didn't you know, she's in a mental hospital.' They were speechless with embarrassment. This was not an isolated or extreme attitude to mental illness. Numerous people still think it is something to be ashamed of, and psychological problems are regarded with fear, scorn or misapprehension.

Some of my own friends tried to persuade me not to take up the subject, saying it would prove too depressing. How wrong they were! Others welcomed this study and encouraged me by their stimulating questions. Many people have been glad of the opportunity for informal discussion of the problems they meet, and what follows is largely the fruit of these meetings.

Despite an encouraging change in the prevailing public attitude to mental illness, and increased understanding of the effect of psychological stress, suspicion and prejudice still prevent many people from seeking the help they need. This was so with Jim Brown. He liked his job, which he had held for five years, but lately he seemed to be getting careless. Instead of sitting at his desk and getting on with the work before him, he was becoming more and more fidgety.

He would open and close the windows several times a day, and was easily distracted. Every time the phone rang, or anything else interrupted his concentration, he would rearrange his files and shuffle his papers before he could start work again. The slightest sound made him jump. He was easily upset and felt very ashamed that he could no longer hide his growing irritability.

In three months he had changed from an efficient, energetic colleague who was easy to get on with, to one who was moody and increasingly unpredictable. His boss told him to pull up his socks. His friends persuaded him to see his doctor. When he got worse and the doctor advised him to see a psychiatrist his family were very upset. Everyone was relieved when he suddenly developed acute appendicitis and was rushed to hospital with a 'respectable' illness.

Most people with a bad appendix welcome the help of a surgeon. Many of them, especially if they have strong religious convictions, do not wish to see a psychiatrist when it is their nerves whch are causing the trouble. The view that psychological and bodily ills are in completely different categories where the agencies for treatment and healing are concerned is a mistaken and illogical one. We are told that Jesus Christ healed every disease, and it is reasonable to assume that this includes emotional as well as physical illnesses. We cannot, therefore, simply on Christian grounds, accept modern advances in treating bodily ills and reject those that deal with our mental and emotional troubles.

This confusion stems from failure to realize that mental processes and spiritual life are two distinct (although interrelated) aspects of a person. Thinking of them both as being one and the same thing limits our understanding of ourselves, and where illness is concerned it causes unnecessary additional suffering. Minor mental upsets, like so many physical ones, usually resolve with the passage of time alone, or in conjunction with simple home remedies. When they do not, medical help should be obtained.

Reluctance to seek help when it is necessary often arises from lack of understanding that the mind, like the body, has many different aspects. Each of these aspects needs to work in close co-operation with all the others for full health to be maintained. The totality of the mind (and especially its emotional, 'feeling' aspect) will both affect and be affected by the degree of efficiency with which the body works.

Emotional factors exert a profound influence on the body through special nerve pathways from the brain and spinal cord to the various organs, which in turn send messages back into the central nervous system. There is a continuous silent exchange of signals between mind and body. A signal from one of them brings about an alteration in the activity of the other, which then sends back a message that this has taken place.

Emotional and bodily factors play a considerable part in determining spiritual responsiveness at any given time. Because the various activities which go to make up a full and complete life cannot occur in isolation from each other, the health and efficiency of the body, together with the general emotional state of the individual, are bound to affect the level of spiritual awareness. They affect it, but they cannot be said to determine or actually control it.

Despite the fact that there is much in common between them, we must remember that none of the various mental functions should be regarded as completely identical with spiritual life. Both mind and body are subject to decreasing efficiency in old age. Mental processes may become disorganised or suspended but it is part of Christian belief that spiritual life survives these changes, and continues after death.

The spirit and mind of man are two different dimensions of his life. They tend to be regarded as one and the same thing simply because neither can be touched, handled, and seen, as the body can. Both belong to the realm of thought and feeling, and all too often both defy our wills. Broadly speaking, with our minds we respond to the world we live in and with our spirits we respond to the God who made us.

People often say that a Christian should not have a nervous breakdown. This statement needs careful thought, because it is a serious claim to make. Although conscious attitudes are affected by beliefs, actual mental processes and mechanisms of the unconscious mind are not altered. St Paul clearly teaches, and experience confirms, that the 'old nature' continues to be active throughout natural life. To suggest that a particular spiritual experience, or adherence to a set of beliefs, can protect a predisposed individual from breaking down under stress is both cruel and dangerous.

To state that no follower of Jesus Christ should ever experience disabling nervous distress is a sweeping generalisation. It is cruel because it implies that if he does do so his spiritual life must be responsible through some fault of his own. For too long it has been assumed that mental or emotional illness is a sign of spiritual and moral inferiority. In fact, whatever connection exists between such illness and the spiritual state of the person it is certainly not a simple one of direct cause and effect.

The statement is dangerous because it may prevent someone from seeking treatment. This is especially important in depressive illness, when it is not unknown for a severely affected person to kill not only himself but his family also. These tragic deaths can so easily be prevented by early medical treatment of the depression. In other conditions, where treatment produces a less speedy and dramatic recovery, the worst of the suffering can quickly be relieved.

Some people, when they do decide to seek treatment, specify that they will only do so from another Christian. They do not realise that there are relatively few valid reasons for such a stipulation. A young married man wrote and asked me to recommend a psychiatrist in his part of the country. He was suffering from feelings of inferiority, shyness and fear of meeting people so that he did not even like going to church.

He said, 'You will understand why I need to tell a Christian about these things. I don't think a non-Christian doctor would understand how important church life is to Christians.' Perhaps not, but he would certainly be familiar with the symptoms and know how to treat them.

A disabled football player eager to get back to the pitch does not say he will only consult a doctor who understands the intricacies of the sport. He goes to the one best qualified to deal with his injury.

Too often when someone suffers from a minor psychiatric disability it is assumed that he will need the services of either the doctor *or* the parson. It is seldom a case of either/or, for usually the distinctive help of both will be required if maximum benefit is to be achieved. During any period of emotional upheaval a person is likely to question most or all of his previously accepted values and beliefs. This leaves him a prey to every kind of doubt and uncertainty, but it is often a necessary prelude to improvement.

He is especially vulnerable when some of his beliefs have been adopted to meet a psychological need. For instance, people who dread meeting others and lack confidence in themselves are often attracted to Churches with an exceptionally narrow outlook. They may fervently believe it is 'wrong' to attend certain social functions, but fundamentally they stay away in order to avoid meeting people rather than because of any principle involved.

Similarly, others consider they should never go to the cinema, while some think it is a waste of time to read a novel of any kind. This rigid view is adopted as a protection from contemporary problems, rather than as part of a consistent code of conduct. Because they do not expose themselves to new ideas they can avoid making their own decisions about the way to live.

When the underlying reasons for such a limited outlook are gradually explored, the person begins to feel all at sea. He loses his false security. It is good that he should do so but he needs an understanding and enlightened approach to help him through this dark, distressing experience. He will go through much heart-searching before he can re-establish his faith on a more mature and biblical basis.

This can be a refining and creative process if adequate guidance is given in both psychological and spiritual matters. Psychiatrist and parson need to work together more. Unfortunately, psychiatrists do not always recognise the existence of spiritual problems, parsons are sometimes unsympathetic to psychiatric ones, and both professions tend to mistrust each other.

A psychiatrist cannot, by virtue of his profession, pronounce on spiritual matters and a parson should not try to be an amateur psychiatrist. Mutual confidence is necessary if they are to be fully effective in their work. Neither can deal with only one aspect of man, and ignore the rest. Both are dealing with the whole person, but from different standpoints and with different resources. Psychiatrists need to know and understand more about the work and calling of parsons, who in turn need a greater appreciation of emotional problems, if they are to establish the necessary confidence in each others' integrity.

Rather than being given special immunity from psychological stress, as some people seem to claim, those who take their religion seriously can expect to face hazards that do not confront other people. This is because their standards are high and they are exposed to many subtle forms of pressure on all sides. A new dimension has entered their lives. Instead of thinking only of themselves and their own interests they will at times be subject to the pull of opposing forces.

There is no valid reason why anyone should expect to be delivered from distress of mind at times or in circumstances when he would not claim such exemption from distress of his body. It is not the mind (in isolation) nor the body (in isolation) but the *entire person* which is redeemed by Jesus Christ. Although the finite part of man (his body together with the brain and mind controlling it) participates in the living experience of Christ, that process is not completed on this earth. While it is incomplete suffering is inescapable.

It is surely presumptuous to claim deliverance from something which Christ did not shrink from facing, in full measure and on our behalf. We are told that in Gethsemane He began to be sorrowful and troubled. It is clear that He suffered strong mental torment, and it was during this agony of mind that He received special strength to enable Him to face the full impact of His situation. He did not turn away from suffering, but when He continued steadfast *despite it* He received strength to carry on to the end.

There is a way for weakness to become strength. This happens when that weakness, whatever it may be, is consciously accepted and given over to Jesus Christ. This giving must be a deliberate act, undertaken with expectation of its efficacy. Many people find it helpful to pray audibly about this, because they then have to be quite definite about their intentions and their requests. Having committed the weakness, and the worry about it, to Christ, one must not sit back and expect to feel different. It is only as one gets on with living, and does the difficult things, that strength to do them comes. The power of God only becomes available as one draws upon it in the time of need; it is not given in advance.

Christ told the apostle Paul, 'My power is made perfect in weakness,' and Paul commented, 'For the sake of Christ, then, I am content with weaknesses, insults, hardships, persecutions, and calamities; for when I am weak then I am strong' (2 Cor. 12. 9, 10 RSV). He knew fear and trembling, uncertainty and loneliness, as well as physical pain and suffering. He was actually grateful for his weakness because it was through this that the power of God became evident to him. It was also more obvious to others than it would have been had he had confidence in his own ability.

We are promised strength to enable us to cope with difficulties when we could not do so in our own strength. The difficulty is not altered, but our approach to it is. Too often we ask God to remove what is troubling us, and to provide us with a ready escape route. Rather we should seek from Him the courage we need to face each crisis. Some will need to go further and seek the causes in themselves which make them liable to recurrent crises.

Much nervous illness is caused by tension within the personality. We must seek to discover and remove the root of this tension so that the energy it consumes may be used for more productive activities. To assume that such illnesses can only be due to spiritual failure is to overlook other equally vulnerable areas. It also falsely assumes that there can be only one reason for the condition. Neither of these assumptions is true. We must look at other possible reasons more closely if we are not to miss something else of importance to the whole person.

2

WHY A BREAKDOWN?

Joan W. had always been rather shy. At school her work was a good average but she was inclined to be timid. She maintained her place near the top of the 'B' stream and then followed her more adventurous friend to a job in the city fifty miles away. Homesickness nearly made her give it up, but after moving into a hostel she made more friends, settled down and began to enjoy life.

When her boy-friend joined the forces without telling her, she was stunned and bewildered. He visited her once but it was not long before even his letters stopped and she realised he had lost interest in her. She seemed to be getting over this blow remarkably well and then one day she was knocked down on a pedestrian crossing. She was taken to hospital with minor injuries and allowed to go home the same day, but six months later she was off work with a nervous breakdown. Her parents told their friends that she had never properly recovered from the road accident.

People often say that they have never been the same since

they had a certain operation, witnessed a particular incident, or received a bad shock. Both they and their relatives may believe that without this one event they would never have had any nervous trouble, but a nervous breakdown does not occur because of a single isolated event. It is the end result of several factors which interact on each other in a complex way.

Whether or not a person has a breakdown depends partly on the constitution he inherits at conception, partly on the strength or weakness of the personality he develops, and partly on the type and timing of any adverse circumstances he meets. Also, of course, his state of body and mind at the time he is confronting a crisis are always important in determining how well he is able to cope with it.

It is the sum of all these varied influences, inherited and acquired, which determines whether his combined physical, emotional, and spiritual resources will enable him to make a constructive adjustment to his circumstances.

Any physical accident or illness can, and usually does, produce a psychological effect. It not only hurts, it also worries, frightens, angers or depresses the sufferer. Certain illnesses cause specific changes in mental outlook and processes. These changes give rise to less worried concern if they are recognised as a usual, and fortunately temporary, part of the original physical illness.

Influenza and other fevers are frequently followed by depression, but only rarely is it more than a passing nuisance. Tropical illnesses have a more severe effect, and the climate may be an additional burden to the foreigner, often prolonging the general debility. Alterations in glandular activity also exert a profound effect on the mind and emotions. Disorders of the thyroid gland, when it works either too hard or not hard enough, produce notable mental changes but they quickly return to normal as soon as the biochemistry of the body is corrected.

In minor nervous troubles physical illness and pressure from the environment are not as important, generally speaking, as conflicting standards and impulses arising from within the individual. When external stress, such as business, financial or domestic worries, appears to trigger off an illness it can only do so if the soil (the person) is right for the seed (the stress) to germinate. If the soil is not suitable the seed will fail to grow.

Mental illness can perhaps be better understood if it is seen as the reaction to stress of a particular individual, rather than as a specific response to a given situation. When someone gets ill with pneumonia it is because he succumbs to a definite germ. His illness is the result of the way his lungs in particular, and his body in general, have reacted to the foreign organism that has invaded his system from outside.

Many people are exposed to similar pneumonia-producing germs, but not all become ill through them. Those who remain well either have lungs that are so healthy the germs are unable to get a hold of them, or if they begin to take hold the body defends itself vigorously and the germs are quickly rendered harmless. Similarly, every person has to meet emotional stresses and strains many times during his life, but some have a greater capacity and resilience with which to meet them.

Some people are unable to function satisfactorily when they meet the normal difficulties of everyday life. They break down and become ill in situations where other people might do no more than show slight signs of discomfort. Such people are the psychological cripples of life, in the same way as a person who gets disabling bronchitis every time there is a fog may be called a respiratory cripple.

One gets ill every time the amount of dust and water in the air becomes too much for his lungs to cope with. The other breaks down when the emotional demands upon him exceed his capacity to meet them. It is then necessary to lessen the immediate demands he has to cope with, and at the same time help him to develop a greater capacity for dealing with a more normal amount of stress in the future.

People react to apparently similar circumstances in very different ways, depending on their temperament and personality. Temperament is inherited. We are born with the capacity to develop certain trends that will shape the rest of our lives, certain definite ways of appreciating and responding to our environment. Also, we are born without certain other traits and tendencies that other people are endowed with. Although an untrained eye can see no difference between an egg from a Buff Orpington hen and one from a Rhode Island Red, the first egg will produce a chick that will unmistakably become a Buff Orpington while the second can become only a Rhode Island Red and no other variety of hen.

We cannot alter the basic material of which we are made, we can only use it more, or less, completely. Trying to become something which nature never intended us to be is a misuse of our inheritance. A Buff Orpington chick can never become a Rhode Island Red hen, however hard it tries. Indeed, the harder it tries the less efficient and contented it will be as a Buff Orpington.

A nervous breakdown is likely to occur when a person has endeavoured to develop characteristics that nature never intended him to have. In trying to do so he will inevitably have neglected to develop resources that do belong to his given temperament. Only truly innate characteristics, properly developed and well integrated, are sufficient to meet and master the crises of life.

To emphasise or under-employ any one aspect of mind will lead to its becoming either under- or over-developed compared with the rest. The intellect that we think and reason with, the will that determines and holds us to a course of action, and the emotional 'feeling' part of us all need to be developed as far as possible. They must also work harmoniously together if full health and maturity are to be achieved.

In Western culture and education the intellectual aspect of mind is over-valued. Because of this it is sometimes over-developed at the expense of other aspects of the personality. The equally important, though more intangible, contributions that are made by intuition, feeling and sensory appreciation tend to be relatively ignored.

Some people are so intellectual that they seem to be without any feeling, they are insensitive to anything other than ideas. Others respond to every new situation with whatever feeling it first arouses in them. Emotion rather than intellect dominates their reactions. They may be, and often are, highly intelligent but they have not learnt to use their intellect in regulating their own responses to life. Another form of one-sidedness is seen in those who always react intuitively. Their response to a situation depends more on its private significance than on reflective thought or spontaneous feeling.

All of these responses are normal ones. Usually an individual who relies on one of them as his initial reaction learns to modify and supplement it by using one or more of the others as well. It is only when one response is relied on to the exclusion of the others that inner tension develops. The wider the range of responses available to a person, the more stable he will be.

When the various aspects of the mind are each developed to a different degree there is bound to be disharmony. They have become, as it were, out of step with each other. Someone whose differing mental functions have grown unevenly will inevitably show signs of tension and stress. To expect otherwise is like expecting children of three, seven and twelve years old to play happily together all the time. They cannot do so because the level of development each has arrived at is so very different.

We must now consider why some people only develop their personalities to a limited extent, and others try to become what nature never intended them to be. Personality can be defined as the individual method a person develops for meeting and adjusting to the varying situations he encounters. In a healthy person it is a continually developing, living, dynamic, harmonious totality of conscious and unconscious attitudes.

Children tend to acquire by imitation the characteristics they admire in older or highly respected people. In very young children this is done quite unconsciously but later it is sometimes deliberate. These models are first and foremost the parents, later older brothers and sisters, teachers and friends. At a still later stage youngsters turn to leaders of their favourite preoccupation, 'pop' stars, sportsmen and other national figures.

Looking out of the window one day I saw Ronald, aged four, strut down the garden alone and stand surveying the cabbage-patch. He had exactly the same stance and expression seen in his father, and his father's father, every fine week-end. Less obvious but just as accurate is the taking over of inner standards and habits of thought. The young schoolboy watches closely the habits of his favourite teacher; in trying to learn his methods of working he also picks up many small incidental habits of thought and behaviour.

Children take over the standards and values of their parents and then test them out as they grow up. Some are found to be helpful and to fit in with what the child himself experiences as he experiments with life. These will be retained in his own emerging system. Others will be modified or discarded gradually if they are found to be consistently at variance with life as he finds it. This assimilation, modification or rejection of parental attitudes proceeds continuously (unless a crippling neurosis intervenes) until maturity is reached.

A growing child should have the maximum opportunity to meet and mingle with people of all ages, interests and outlooks in order to further his own development. He requires the stimulus of others to give him the example, the pattern, the ideals which will develop his own latent abilities. When he can identify with a person who possesses what is only latent in himself, this quality will be activated into growth.

Identification and unconscious imitation are not confined to the very young, as Dr Paul Brand startlingly discovered one day in India. Pioneer in reconstructive surgery of the hands and feet of leprosy victims, he watched one of his registrars examine a patient in the Christian Medical College, Vellore. 'He stared at the registrar who, while asking a rather embarrassing question of the patient, had one eyebrow raised and, head tilted to one side, was peering out under his eyebrows with a little twisted half smile.

' "However did you get that expression on your face?" he asked. 'It's the exact image of my old professor in London."

'The house surgeons laughed. "That's your face, sir," one of them said.

'Paul was amazed and shocked. Was it possible that in those past years he had absorbed, not only the surgical teaching, but the little routine details of bedside manner, right down to the position of the eyebrows and the twist of the lips and the stance beside the bed?

' "Then what am *I* passing on?" he thought with profound

24

concern. "From where have I received it, and how far is it going?" [1]

Every individual's pattern of life is largely determined by various inner needs and the necessity to satisfy them in one way or another. There are physiological, that is bodily, needs like hunger, thirst, sex, sleep and the maintenance of a moderately even body temperature. There are also psychological requirements like the need for affection, approval, companionship and security; and there are equally fundamental spiritual needs.

These include the necessity to find a meaning and purpose in life, to establish a personal identity and to have a creative apprehension of an external, eternal power. Anything which prevents the satisfaction of any one of these needs results in mounting tension. When the ensuing discomfort reaches a certain level, which varies from person to person, some action to reduce it becomes imperative.

Sometimes it is possible to reduce the urgency of a need, as for instance when previously almost overwhelming sleepiness is dispelled by the overriding interest of a late TV show. When satisfaction of the need can neither be delayed nor reduced, and appropriate means of satisfying it are not available, substitute ones are sought. For instance, over-eating is commonly an attempt to compensate for unsatisfactory interpersonal relationships, and one reason that some young people take advantage of the current availability of addictive drugs is

[1] Dorothy Clarke Wilson, *Ten Fingers for God* (Hodder and Stoughton).

the vain hope of finding some meaning and stimulation in their purposeless lives.

What action is taken is not governed by deliberate, conscious choice. It will be influenced, to a greater or lesser extent, by unconscious needs and pressures. The Christian's aim is that all natural appetites should be his servant rather than his master, so that they can be fully employed to the glory of God. For this to be possible they must be as much as possible under his conscious scrutiny and control. When natural appetites are not so scrutinised it is because of some difficulty in development which has caused them to become isolated from the main stream of his life.

If a child's attempt to satisfy a basic need constantly meets with disapproval and he cannot find any acceptable alternative, the whole conflict situation is likely to be pushed out of conscious awareness. Because it is insoluble it is intolerable. The need itself, and the feelings associated with it, does not cease to exist. It will continue to be a source of tension but, because it is unconscious, its true origin is hidden from the adult. Many symptoms of nervous illness arise from unsuccessful, or only partially successful, attempts to reduce this tension.

We all like to find an explanation for experiences that we do not understand. Frequently a late supper will be held responsible for a sleepless night, even though on other occasions a larger and later meal has been followed by quick, peaceful slumber. This is because it is so much more tolerable to blame a supposedly indigestible meal, which one can account for, than the unconscious, which one cannot. But the unconscious is a God-given part of ourselves and cannot be ignored or decried just because we do not fully understand this and other disturbances in our lives.

The unconscious is much more than a repository for unruly drives and feelings. It contains all the unrealised potential of the individual, all his latent abilities and talents which are waiting to be utilised. It is a reservoir of creative energy waiting to be tapped. It is one of the many 'members' of the human person. Paul, writing of the importance and inter-dependence of every separate part for the proper functioning of the whole, says, 'God arranged the organs in the body, each one of them, as he chose' (1 Cor. 12. 18 RSV). He goes on to warn against assuming any part of the body to be less valuable to the whole than any other part, for all are needed in their proper place.

We may perhaps liken ourselves to a large onion which, when one starts to explore how it is made, always seems to have another layer beneath the one that is currently being looked at. It is this 'something more than' our outward appearance to others, and 'more than' our own conscious experience of ourselves, that constitute the unconscious. There are differing hypotheses about how the unconscious works, but we cannot because of this ignore its existence.

At the beginning of this century it was thought that one particularly harmful event, especially if it were dramatic, was sufficient to cause certain nervous states. For instance, a woman walking alone down the street became suddenly paralysed on hearing distant gunfire, although she received no physical injury from it. Further experience of such cases showed that there was always a far more personal reason for the symptom than just 'shock'. To produce such a profound effect the shock must have had a particular meaning of a threatening nature to the individual concerned.

The gunfire reminded her that her father had recently been posted to the local unit. Although she had done nothing wrong, she knew that he would strongly disapprove of the friend she was on her way to visit. The cause of the paralysis was certainly not the distant gunfire, nor can it be dismissed as guilty conscience.

The real cause of her paralysis became apparent when her relationship with her parents was understood. Their influence in her life was so strong that she found it difficult to make a life of her own, or to choose her own friends. She knew that she could not retain her father's approval if she persisted with that friendship, but she could not bear to part with either, and the conflict within literally paralysed her.

Today it is generally accepted that the quality of personal relationships formed in childhood, and the repeated pattern of influences encountered, are of crucial importance in shaping later reactions. The seeds of neurosis are sown when the values absorbed from the environment, and particularly from misguided parental pressures, conflict with the individual's own growing experience of himself and others.

One mother, hoping to make her sensitive son less upset by criticism, deliberately taught him to repeat, 'Sticks and stones will break my bones, but words will never hurt me.' She made him repeat it again and again whenever he came home from nursery school with some tale of woe. He said it fiercely, trying to convince himself that his feelings were not hurt, but this did violence to the facts. Denial does not equip a child to deal with distress.

That teaching implanted in him the idea that whenever he was upset at being teased, he came short of his mother's standard and was therefore 'bad'. He came to regard himself as an inferior being, and all emotions as 'bad' things to experience. Because of this much that should have been a positive, creative force in his life became instead a source of embarrassing tension in later years.

The most frequent source of conflict is still, despite all the attention given to it, in the whole field of sexuality. No other activity, interest and outlet of which man is capable can be so far-reaching in its effect, yet this always remains an exceptionally personal and individual matter. Whether or not a person accepts the challenge it presents, and how he comes to terms with this great instinctive force, will determine a large part of his character. It will greatly affect how he conducts himself in every situation. It will determine both his confidence in himself and the way he relates to other people, for the two are indissolvably linked together.

In trying to understand what may have caused a nervous breakdown we have to consider not one but many factors. It is the total situation of present circumstances in the light of past events that proves too much for the person concerned, rather than one isolated event. A straw may break the back of the proverbial camel, but only when it is added to an already considerable load or placed on an already overstrained animal.

We must be sensitive to the feelings and susceptibilities of every person with whom we come in contact. When we think of the other person rather than ourself, and try to understand him from his point of need, we shall be unlikely to add that last straw which precipitates a breakdown. And we shall be obeying the rule of love expounded and exemplified by Jesus Christ.

It is regrettable that some Christian teaching, badly presented, encourages a destructive self-attitude and so makes it more, rather than less, likely that a predisposed individual will break down under stress. This happens particularly when there is an incomplete and one-sided presentation of sin and condemnation without a correspondingly vigorous proclamation of the grace and mercy of God.

There is often need for more stress on sin as a *collective* as well as an individual condition, and on God's love freely given on an *individual* as well as on a collective basis. People with a self-condemnatory bias need to be shown the dominance of the love of God. Law and judgment are an essential part of Christian teaching, but only a part. When these aspects fill a person's thoughts to the exclusion of grace and mercy they result in a very inadequate religion. Love, not law, is the key to full spiritual development.

The good news that every individual is a valuable and

worthwhile *person* to God does not always get enough emphasis. Systematic teaching of the whole counsel of God contains the answer to all man's spiritual needs and, wisely applied, it reduces this source of inner tension. Spiritual maturity will render a person able to cope with pressing psychological problems better than he could without this source of strength. It will not solve his psychological problems, nor remove the necessity to deal with them by psychological means.

3

THE INFLUENCE OF SEX

At thirty, Bill was still devoting all his leisure time and energy to the pursuit of a higher academic qualification. He was a conscientious worker and a loyal colleague, who made a good deputy but lacked the originality and powers of leadership necessary to head a department of his own. His sense of humour was buried deep beneath a load of cares; life for him was essentially a question of 'getting on'. Even his hobbies were pursued with a seriousness and grim intensity that prevented him obtaining any real relaxation.

He played tennis regularly and fanatically, always choosing a partner of equal or slightly higher standard than himself so that he could continually improve his game. He had never joined a club, ostensibly because that would involve too much 'waste of time' in waiting his turn for a game, but there was a more fundamental reason. The social side of club life scared him. This fact he successfully hid from himself until he was forced to reappraise his goals when, for the third time, he failed to gain promotion.

He discovered that his constant preoccupation with getting on in life was keeping him away from living. Lonely and dissatisfied with himself, he had not recognised the deep urge for a life partner. Recognising and satisfying this fundamental urge would involve a side of his nature that he had come to regard as the enemy of success, and little short of evil in itself.

The opposite approach to life was shown by Eric when he was in his early twenties. He had had a number of girl-friends, and with several of them a full sexual relationship was established. Soon after his engagement was announced he found to his great dismay that he had become impotent.

Bill had been alarmed by his developing sexuality and had tried to deny and disown its striving by pouring all his attention into his career. Eric had tried to achieve a sense of power and importance through physical gratification. Both Eric and Bill had been unable to accept the full responsibilities of adult manhood, but they showed it in different ways.

These attitudes and other sexual difficulties can be explained by childhood experiences. In our society it seems to be inevitable that some degree of guilt about sexuality will be conveyed to children as they grow up. The standards, attitudes and expectations of society exert pressure on parents, so that however well they deal with their children's behaviour at home, they are unlikely to entirely escape embarrassment when dealing with much the same questions and behaviour in front of other people. Although many parents have learnt not to punish a child when he starts playing with or commenting upon his sexual organs, they are unlikely to express open approval of such activity.

When every other new discovery and activity is praised and this exciting one is ignored, the difference in parental attitudes is quickly appreciated by the child. A sensitive one is likely to equate accurately the absence of comment with some measure of disapproval or doubt. Also of course the anatomical proximity of the excretory and genital organs means that the 'don't touch', 'dirty', 'unclean' attitudes to the former are very easily extended to the latter as well.

Anatomical differences between the two sexes are of course immediately apparent at birth. There are undoubtedly two classes of citizens, two classes of people—not rich or poor, good or bad, black or white, wanted or unwanted, lovely or shameful, admired or despised—but quite simply male or female. A young child not only learns that he is a boy or she is a girl but also develops an attitude towards himself, as a result of various subtle cues picked up from his parents. This attitude is summed up by one adjective from several of the above opposites, for instance he may feel that he is unwanted and despised because he is so often naughty.

If he is fortunate in his early relationships, and knows without a doubt that he is loved and wanted by his parents, he will have a predominant feeling of goodness, rightness and acceptability that he will apply to the whole range of his personal experience. If he is not so fortunate he may, in his mind, split off some of his experiences and the part of his body with which he appreciates them, and regard these as bad and unacceptable, or at best undesirable.

There are many ways in which the confidence that a child has in himself, and particularly in his sexual role, can be unwittingly undermined. If on grazing his knee and being told to be a good (brave, strong) boy and not cry, he does not manage to stop crying, a more lasting hurt may occur if he comes to regard himself as 'bad' (cowardly, weak) because he could not do so. This adjective 'bad' is then specifically linked with the 'boy' aspect of himself. He has not behaved as a good (brave, strong) boy is expected to behave so he feels that the 'boy' in him must be bad, cowardly and weak. Such an attitude will make him timid and unsure of himself.

An unjustified discrimination between the sexes, or on the other hand a failure to acknowledge that there is any difference, can also impart a sense of sexual inferiority. When parents loudly insist that their girls are treated the same as the boys, especially in the matter of educational opportunity and personal freedom, this unintentionally but very effectively makes the girls feel inferior. They are not being treated as individuals, but in comparison to boys. The very insistence on equality implies the assumption of an innate lack of it.

Childhood experience largely determines how the pressing demands of emerging sexual impulses and feelings are dealt with at puberty. The relationship between the two parents, and the regard with which the child holds them both, will be of great importance. If they are genuinely and evidently happy with each other, and enjoy their special relationship together,

35

then growing up to be like mother or father will be something to desire, welcome and encourage. If on the other hand the parental relationship is not good, or the child has difficulty in getting on with either or both of his parents, then attaining adult status and responsibilities will be viewed with apprehension.

Children sense a strained atmosphere, and are affected by it, without giving it conscious, deliberate thought. Because they are consistently excluded from their parents' sexual relationship, it is not surprising that they tend to blame this for any atmosphere of bitterness or anger between the parents. If the child then equates the sexual act only with aggression and hostility he is very likely to turn away from and be afraid of his own developing sexuality. He will feel that it is something to ward off and deny as long as possible, rather than a natural development to be encouraged.

A child needs a good relationship with both parents if his development is to be as smooth and complete as possible. He needs to be able to identify himself with the parent of his own sex, for if that parent does not give him an attractive example of what being an adult entails, he will have no positive incentive to grow up. He will not wish to do so and will remain immature in outlook. The resulting insecurity will make him more dependent upon and emotionally bound to the parent from whose attitudes he most needs to emancipate himself. It is the pathological *attitudes* of the parent rather than the *actual* parent from which such a person needs to extricate himself if he is to become a stable, independent adult.

The parent of the opposite sex to the child also has an important part to play in his emotional development, for he will be the prototype of any future sexual partner. If the example given is an attractive one it will be an encouragement to reach out, but if it is a forbidding one it will be a barrier to further development.

It is the search for a partner which drives those who recognise their need out of the immediate family protection and into the wider world. This makes the individual more (but never completely) independent. At the same time it opens the way to enrichment rather than weakening of the family by opening it to the influence of new interests, new ideas, new ways and fresh horizons. Erotic urges are neither a curse to be endured nor a panacea to be indulged in at all times. They are a manifestation of normal, healthy life which affords a special satisfaction and pleasure while subserving other purposes also.

The body, with its appetites and passions, was regarded by ancient Greek philosophers as an evil tomb which imprisoned and restricted the soul in its search for pure knowledge. Plato, in his account of Socrates' last hours, wrote: 'For the body is a source of endless trouble to us by reason of the mere requirement of food; and is liable also to diseases which overtake and impede us in the search after true being; it fills us full of loves, and lusts, and fears, and fancies of all kinds, and endless foolery, and in fact, as men say, takes away from us the power of thinking at all.' This is an exaggerated regard for intellect, and an undervaluation of bodily needs and pleasures.

Any exaggeration tends to result in a reactionary swing to the opposite direction. Another philosophical school, that of Epicurus in the third century BC, laid the foundation for just such a reversal of values. The Epicureans taught that pleasure alone is the highest good, and although they stressed mental rather than sensual pleasures, a sect arose which misconstrued this teaching and encouraged every form of licence and excess. Neither attitude is confined to older civilisations in other lands.

The Victorians decried (when they did not deny) the value of bodily gratification, with the result that today it is again over-emphasised. D. H. Lawrence represented the modern age when he wrote: 'I believe the life of the body is a greater reality than the life of the mind,' and so he perpetuates the artificial separation of the body from the rest of human experience.

The Christian view on this matter neither exalts nor execrates the body, but sees it always in relation to its Creator. It sees the body as of vital but not sole importance; an essential part of man's being which must be properly used but not abused. This attitude was summed up by the apostle Paul when he wrote: ' "All things are lawful for me," but not all things are helpful. "All things are lawful for me," but I will not be enslaved by anything . . . Do you not know that your body is a temple of the Holy Spirit within you, which you have from God? You are not your own; you were bought with a price. So glorify God in your body' (1 Cor. 6. 12, 19, 20 RSV). The emphasis is on God, not self, and we are told to glorify Him

38

in the body. One cannot do that if one neglects it on the one hand or over-indulges it on the other.

Long ago Luther pointed out that Jesus, who is sinless, had a body but the devil, who is the originator of sin, is without a body. The tremendous pleasure which can (quite legitimately) be obtained from the body has made many people neglect to cultivate it for fear that they will become its slave. The dangers of excess are sometimes emphasised in such an unbalanced way that anything at all pleasurable arouses a feeling of guilt, while everything that is difficult or dreary is seen as a virtue. What a travesty of our faith, what utter mockery that is!

Our bodies belong to the world of nature, they are part of its rich furnishing given for our enjoyment. Anyone who ignores his body for fear that its demands will become unmanageable will suffer as a result. A mature person is free to satisfy or deny these demands according to his judgment of the circumstances. Control like this, consciously exercised, is called suppression and must not be confused with repression.

Repression is banishing unacceptable ideas, impulses or wishes to the unconscious. This does not get rid of them entirely; they continue to exert an influence but can now do so only indirectly. Behaviour is then determined by unconscious forces rather than by conscious control. Repression is psychologically harmful because it limits the free choice of the individual.

A young child is an inquisitive being who learns and develops as the result of his own exploration. The first thing he will explore is his own body and he soon realises that gentle friction of certain sensitive parts will induce a state of generalised pleasure. The mouth is the first area to be discovered and used in this way; when the breast or bottle is not available many infants resort to thumb sucking when they are in need of comfort. Soon the anal region and at a later date the genitals are found to be sensitive areas, appropriate stimulation of them inducing a similar state of generalised physical pleasure.

In infancy this simple pleasure is not associated with erotic thoughts or desires, for the appropriate higher nervous centres are not sufficiently developed. Much confusion has come from applying adult standards, desires and reasoning to immature bodies and minds. During childhood mental imagery and phantasy gradually become associated with masturbation and although the opposite sex have not yet begun to acquire special significance it is probable that, as Havelock Ellis puts it, 'the psychic condiment of forbidden fruit may be added to its enjoyment.'[1]

The literal meaning of masturbation is genital stimulation with the hand but it has been extended to cover any method of using friction to produce pleasure from the genital area. Around puberty similar pleasurable sensations can be aroused by appropriate thoughts alone. As development proceeds more interest is taken in, and stimulation received from, contacts with the opposite sex. It is not until this time that masturbation begins to be associated with and to pass over into adult sexual activity. When erotic stimulation comes from contact with or

[1] Havelock Ellis, *The Psychology of Sex* (Pan).

ideas about the opposite sex it is being obtained from a bio-logically appropriate object. This is the normal sequence of development unless guilt or fear hamper (and sometimes totally prevent) this transition.

Doubt and uncertainty about oneself become prominent during adolescence. There is frequently a more or less passing feeling of being unloved and unwanted. If excessive this can all too easily make the adolescent feel that he must be essentially unlovable and so his despair about himself is deepened. One way of obtaining relief and reassurance is through mastur-bation, and when used in this way it becomes a substitute satisfaction.

The physical tension which accompanies many diverse emo-tions can be relieved by this means. It is not a desirable method because it does not affect the underlying situation. Although the physical tension is released, the result is only temporary because the emotional problem remains. It is not the act itself that is harmful but the use to which it is put.

Masturbation used to be called self-abuse. It is still often regarded with abhorrence although such a moralistic attitude tends to prolong rather than curtail its use. It is a normal result of the sexual impulse when aroused in the physical absence of an appropriate biological object, and it frequently occurs spontaneously during sleep. Those who habitually and preferentially resort to it after adolescence need help in finding more appropriate and constructive ways of resolving their emotional difficulties.

We have seen that a child can very easily be made to feel

guilty about his sexuality, and where there is guilt there is frequently fear. A combination of these two emotions underlies all sexual difficulties and deviations. Whatever form it takes (and there are many) perversion is a manifestation of arrested development.

Any act that is divorced from its proper purpose is a perversion. Specifically, in sexual matters this means any behaviour which replaces the desire for sexual intercourse with a physically mature partner of the opposite sex. Because the word perversion is associated with condemnatory moral judgment it will be avoided and the more neutral word deviation (with its rather wider meaning) used instead.

Many objects, activities and phantasies may be substituted for, or added to, the range which normally provokes sexual arousal and terminates in its gratification. Such substitutes arise from emotional conditioning and the way psychological stresses were resolved and dealt with during childhood. They are blind alleys, culs-de-sac off the main road of development; they lead nowhere and so although they give a partial satisfaction to pressing instinctive urges their practice inevitably leaves the sufferer in a state of chronic tension.

There is no conscious and delberate choice in having deviant tendencies. The impulses to unusual actions and the often distressing fantasies to which the deviant is frequently a prey, are as much outside his control as are the nocturnal dreams of any normally adjusted person. A person with unusual tendencies cannot help feeling as he does, or experiencing his particular urges. Whether or not he acts upon these impulses may, because of his general personality problem, be somewhat less under his control than are the heterosexual impulses of the average person.

Homosexuality is seldom adopted deliberately as a perverse way of life. It evolves from attempts to resolve a number of complex and insistent psychological, physiological and sociological pressures. Technically the term includes every degree of attraction for another person of the same sex, from admiration, affection and companionship without obvious erotic arousal or physical contact, through lesser degrees of physical and psychological eroticism right up to a passionate 'love' affair.

Love is written in inverted commas here because no homosexual liaison can ever take the place of a heterosexual relationship. It can never be as complete and satisfying although some see it as the alternative to a lonely and frustrated life.

The positive educational potential of a homosexual attraction must not be overlooked. It may be employed to further the expansion and liberation of the personality rather than for physical gratification. Young people tend to seek out older companions of the same sex in whom they discern qualities which are lacking in themselves. They then make those companions into models upon which their interest centres until they are confident that they themselves possess and can utilise the qualities they admired.

People who fail to make this identification with an adult member of their own sex, normally the parent, suffer from some degree of inferiority in their role as adult men or women.

For this reason they will go on being attracted to members of their own sex, and will feel inadequate in dealings with the opposite one, unless they find someone who can help them to develop further.

Adult homosexual relationships are usually unstable because they are almost invariably disappointing. Partners are changed frequently in the search for fulfilment that is bound to be denied. Only a mature person can really provide what is required, and a mature person is unlikely to reciprocate the relationship in the first place. Usually each partner seeks in the other a substitute for what he feels to be his predominant deficiency; every liaison is an attempt to restore something that is felt to be lacking.

Over-dependent women unconsciously look for someone who will be a mother to them rather than a partner; they desire to be nurtured and provided for without having to contribute actively in return. Women who supply this sought-for protection and guidance do so to satisfy their own repressed maternal impulses. The relationship will therefore be fraught with jealousy and resentment. The dependence of the first and the possessive dominance of the second are both so excessive that they make insatiable demands on each other.

However much they appear to be good for one another initially, after a time they will retard rather than promote growth in each other. If realisation of this state is very nearly a simultaneous occurrence in both partners the break will occasion little emotional upheaval, but frequently there is a 'unilateral declaration of independence' (or more probably a

44

transfer of dependence to someone else). This is likely to spark off an emotional outburst in the one who feels herself to have been rejected and deserted.

Men who always take an excessively masculine partner are seeking, through their identification with him, to make up for the qualities which they feel they lack themselves. Others who are irresistibly drawn to slender, delicately featured men of youthful appearance are likely to have an unconscious fear of women. They do not entirely repress their sexual urges but because of their deep fear they cannot approach a woman. Instead they turn to the nearest safe substitute: a man with feminine characteristics.

According to Fenichel, 'Neurotics are persons whose real actions are blocked.' Although sexual deviants suffer from a distorted pattern of sexual arousal and gratification, their deviant practices are a partial, if sometimes roundabout, outlet. Because these practices afford some measure of satisfaction as well as distress, such people have even more difficulty than 'pure' neurotics in bringing themselves to accept treatment.

Their whole pattern of life, not just one aspect of it, is distorted. Deviant practices are the only method they have found for satisfying emotional needs that are every bit as strong as their physical ones. They see no other way of obtaining companionship, of exchanging something valuable with another person, and of achieving some much needed boost to their low self-esteem.

People whose development has proceeded to a more personally satisfying, and socially satisfactory, level may need to remind themselves that anomalous sexual practices are an attempt to overcome early emotional injuries. A man who has a shortened, undeveloped limb as a result of poliomyelitis (infantile paralysis) arouses sympathy. The individual whose sexual development has been distorted or arrested before maturity is reached has the same claim on our compassion. He requires help in disentangling his fear, and assistance to overcome it, if he is to cope with his personal crisis in a more mature way.

4

VARIOUS TYPES OF DEPRESSION

Rustling the evening paper, Mr Jones sighed deeply as he sat down, noisily impatient. Supper was late again. It had been late several times recently but never before on committee night. What made it worse this time was that Alice no longer seemed to care, and she used to be so particular about getting him out on time. As he looked round the room impatience gave way to concern. Yesterday's newspaper stuffed behind a cushion, a definite film of dust on the bookcase, two unposted letters propped against the clock; not like his Alice at all, he thought.

She had taken to getting up long before him most mornings, although there was no need. The breakfast was frequently either half cooked or badly burnt and she left the conversation to him. As he was usually in a hurry he didn't pay much attention to this at first. In the evenings she would be more talkative, but not really lively, and now he noticed that she was eating very little.

The household jobs got more and more behind; she seemed to have no interest in the television and couldn't even be bothered with her knitting. She was losing weight and forgot so many things that despite her protestations he insisted on her seeing their doctor. She was given some tablets and he saw that she took them regularly. For a time he did more than she did in the house but after a few weeks that was no longer necessary, as she was getting back to her old self again.

A more alarming and dramatic situation arose for Mr Downes. Middle-aged and well established in his profession, he developed a severe eye complaint. To prevent blindness he was given a certain drug which kept the disease under control but caused a deep and dreadful depression. Although he knew the grave risk to his eyesight, Mr Downes actually asked his doctor to stop giving him the drug that was making life so unbearable for him. His depression was so terrible that he preferred to run the risk of going blind, and face the challenge and difficulties that loss of sight would entail, than continue living in such a dejected state. Fortunately it was possible to change his treatment and relieve the depression as well as the eye trouble.

John's case was different again. He had just left College with a good degree and landed a job that he was very keen to get. He had every reason to be on top of the world yet he became unaccountably depressed. At first his friends were concerned and sympathetic, but as time went by and he showed no sign of emerging from his melancholy state, they began to lose patience with him and he with himself.

Some days he felt better than others. He would have more energy and be able to get on with things. But these phases seldom lasted long. He lost interest in his hobbies and was too tired to go out in the evenings any more. He felt worse when he was on his own, yet he could not be bothered with people and was becoming easily irritated over minor matters. Although tired and dispirited he had difficulty in getting off to sleep, and often what sleep he did get would be disturbed by strange dreams. He lost confidence in himself and the plum job he had so much wanted seemed, now that he had got it, an impossible task and an unhappy burden.

Depression is not one illness, it is a symptom indicating that something is wrong, a signal to search out the origin of the disturbance. It can be brought on by many different things and for this reason it is important to obtain medical advice. Sometimes the cause is a physical one, a biochemical deficiency in the body or an unfortunate side-effect of powerful drugs quite properly being taken for another condition. Frequently it is the result of unconscious psychological problems (unacknowledged anger and resentment are common factors). Sometimes it is the effect of unresolved spiritual conflict. What treatment is required will depend on the relative importance of the various causes, which are not mutually exclusive.

When depression is due to physical factors there is usually a systematic go-slow, a diminution of all normal activity. The various bodily appetites are diminished, mental and physical processes become slower and everything is more of an effort. A depressed person is likely to be forgetful; he may lose his sense of values and usually his natural rhythm of sleep is disturbed. Even those who have previously slept well tend to waken earlier. They can still get to sleep easily at night but wake after only a few hours and are unable to get off again.

To a depressed person the most usual and routine tasks seem mountainous, he has no energy and gradually loses interest in his accustomed activities. In severe cases he may neglect himself and his work to the point of slovenliness. This is not due to laziness or lack of moral fibre. The physiology of the body is upset by illness, but all these changes are reversible. Appetite, energy, interest, memory and sleep can all be restored to their former level with the effective forms of treatment now available.

Sometimes the most distressing aspect of this illness is the change which a person experiences in his feelings. He seems to be completely enveloped in a big, black cloud through which there seems to be no way out for him. The present is grim but the future looks darker still. He may falsely interpret this condition as a direct result of his personal actions in the past and may develop a conviction that his suffering is all his own fault: the just judgment for some particular sin. This may be a wholly imaginary incident or a real but trivial one magnified out of all proportion.

When suffering from depression a person often feels that he is letting his employer or his family down, and that he is no longer up to the demands of his job. He may then begin to say that he never was up to it, that his whole life has been based on falsehood. Sometimes he will carry this further and say that the only honourable course is for him to resign immediately. When this is unjustified in the light of his previous record it is wise for employers not to accept his resignation until he has seen his doctor. His action is clearly the result of illness and not something that he would do when well.

Because he feels this way about himself he may even come to attribute his own thoughts to others. At first this will only be an unshakable belief that they agree with his opinions about himself but it often progresses to a conviction that he can actually hear people saying he is wicked. He may also be hounded by a feeling that people are planning to do him some harm as a reprisal for this wickedness.

Another sign of depressive illness is when a person suddenly and uncharacteristically says that he is not worth bothering with, he is far too wicked. He may be convinced that he has ruined himself and others, that he is bringing disgrace to his family, who would be better off without him. He may go further and say that he has committed the 'unforgivable sin' and that there is no hope for him. He feels that destruction is his inevitable end, a just punishment for his 'crimes', and death itself too good for him.

People suffer in this way long before they ever put it into words. When anyone withdraws from contact with others, appears lifeless or becomes too apologetic, medical advice is necessary. Chance expressions of unwarranted guilt, or indications that the person feels exceptionally unworthy, should make his friends realise that he is ill and must be encouraged to see his doctor.

There is always the danger that a seriously depressed person will attempt to commit suicide. He is so utterly despairing, so completely convinced that nothing and nobody can help him, that he cannot help his impulse to self-destruction. He is so sure that he is a burden to others as well as himself that even the strongest moral convictions are sometimes insufficient to withstand such an urge. When questioned sympathetically many people will reluctantly admit that they feel it is no longer worth the struggle to go on living. They are usually quite honest in their assessment of whether or not they are likely to do any harm to themselves. It is imperative to ask them and to take their answer seriously.

The belief that people who talk about suicide never attempt it is quite without foundation. On the contrary, it is usual for them to give some warning of their desperate plight. Relatives and friends must be alert to recognise and heed any warning of impending crisis.

Many people who do not have the energy or initiative to plan their suicide, or whose convictions are firmly against such action, may on sudden impulse take an opportunity if it presents itself. Every sensible precaution must be taken to prevent the opportunity occurring; when tablets are prescribed only one or two days' supply should be left in the possession of the depressed person, the rest being kept by a reliable member of the family. Cupboards should be cleared of all medicines left over from previous illnesses; common household remedies, such as aspirin and its many cousins, must not be overlooked and left lying about the house.

A potentially suicidal person is a sick person and should not be argued with about his condition. To tell him that he is a disgrace to his family and to his Church even to think about such a thing is utterly wrong. It only serves to confirm his prevailing sense of doom and failure; it will make him more rather than less likely to kill himself.

A depressed person cannot be argued out of his distorted view of life, for his attitude is not open to correction by explanation or reason. It is unwise to attempt to alter it with long scriptural exhortations as his state of mind will make him ignore all that is helpful and seize upon any hint of judgment and doom. This view of life will continue until his mind and reasoning powers are restored by medical treatment.

During this period he more than ever needs continued, steady friendship. He needs to feel accepted and must be assured of his place as a valuable and worthwhile member of society. His friends and advisers should remember that his condition is due to illness, not lack of faith or extraordinary sin, and they must encourage him to seek and accept medical treatment. He needs quiet, consistent support and prayer rather than preaching.

Another fact to remember is that sexual desire and responsiveness commonly decrease during a depressive episode. If it is realised that this is part of a much wider alteration in outlook and interest due to illness, much unhappiness will be avoided. Misunderstandings and recriminations are all too likely to occur if the total illness, of which this is but a part, goes unrecognised. The healthy partner may begin to suspect that the patient's loss of interest in him is due to increased interest in someone else. He will then become angry and suspicious, or if of another temperament may himself become depressed and suffer from considerable guilt because of the jealousy aroused: jealousy which he deplores but cannot altogether deny. A whole range of emotions will then arise to complicate the original situation between the partners, unless the loss of sexual interest is seen as part of an illness.

Depressive illness does not necessarily have all the characteristics mentioned, for it comes in many disguises. Mr B. was so agitated that the only way he could stop his legs from shaking was to pace up and down the room as he talked. He could not stay sitting in one chair for long but had to keep jumping up and walking around, returning to his chair with many apologies only to get up again. He complained of various things he felt to be wrong with his body: he said he could not breathe properly, he had terrible headaches and had lost a lot of weight. He did not complain of any change in his mood and he did not think there had been any alteration in his outlook on life.

Despite his great over-activity it was clear from his story and from watching him that he was in fact severely depressed. That is, he had all the evidence of a clinical illness although he did not feel in any way depressed. There was nothing wrong with his lungs and he was not objectively short of breath. All his bodily complaints were quite usual expressions of a depressive illness.

At first Mr B. would not believe this, and he refused the treatment recommended. When he eventually agreed to have it he required persuasion to continue but soon began to improve, and after less than a month he was a different man.

All the aches and pains that he had put up with for more than half a year completely disppeared and he was able to return to work after many months' absence.

It cannot be assumed that depression is necessarily predominantly a spiritual malady just because it is noticed that spiritual interest has declined. Indeed, it is often lost altogether, in keeping with the cessation or diminution of other interests and activities. This, like the others, can be expected to return to its former level as general improvement is achieved with treatment. Of course medical treatment cannot of itself bring about spiritual growth; it can only restore whatever capacity was there before illness robbed the individual of the ability to use it fully.

Some people bear testimony to growth begun during such an illness. They emerge from it with spiritual depth because they have experienced for the first time the truth, reality and relevance of their faith. Only when tested in this or some other way does a person realise that his faith is based not on his own changing feelings but on reliable, objective, steadfast facts. When this is proved by actual personal experience it results in a faith that is stronger and more mature.

Although people do not as a rule complain of having excessive energy, this too can be a warning of impending illness. Fatuous high spirits and pathological over-activity are the most obvious features of changes in mood and behaviour that sometimes alternate with depression. When a person comes for treatment only in the depressed phase it is not unusual to find that he does also have minor episodes of slight over-activity.

To him these seem to be times of increased well-being, although his relatives will sometimes admit, if asked, that there is an element of abnormality about his periodic over-activity.

An over-active phase progressing to real illness can be very trying to relatives and dangerous for the patient. He has more energy than he knows how to employ but it is poorly directed and ill-controlled. He is likely to rush around doing so many things that he never finishes one of them before dashing on to the next. This continues with increasing tempo until he exhausts himself and his resources. His outlook is so coloured by a rosy glow that his judgment is distorted and nothing that he wants, however impractical, seems beyond his reach.

Because of this he will embark on tasks that are far beyond his capacity and he indulges in so many simultaneous grand and hairbrained schemes that his money runs out. Unfortunately this does not deter him, for even large debts appear trifling because of his feeling of omnipotence. This is illness, not wilful extravagance, and he is not properly responsible for his actions while it lasts.

Of a somewhat different order is the depression which occurs in response to adverse circumstances. Some degree of it is to be expected after a bereavement or great disappointment. Personal tragedies naturally result in a feeling of emptiness and can induce a profound sense of loss which leaves the person bewildered and bemused. Depression of this type is easy to understand and sympathise with because its cause is known. It is a period of partial withdrawal from activity and serves to give the sufferer time in which to adjust to his changed circumstances.

There are many other forms of loss which provoke a similar reaction. Their cause, however, is not so apparent and as other people cannot understand what is going on in the sufferer they tend to be unsympathetic. They often say, or at the very least imply, that the depressed person has only to obey the impatient injunction to 'pull himself together' and he will be able to 'snap out of it'. This only makes him feel more alone in his misery, more hopeless and dispirited.

He has not become depressed because he wants to be like this, and he remains depressed because he cannot, rather than because he will not, pull himself out of it. His whole being has reacted in a way that psychiatrists recognise as 'reactive depression'. This is evidence that he is either genuinely unaware of the root of his problem, or that for some reason he is unable to deal with it in a more constructive way. Usually it is both; he is unable to deal with the problem by direct means *because he has not yet defined what it is*. He is torn between two mutually exclusive ideas, one of which is not available to his conscious examination and evaluation.

Whatever the disappointment causing such a depression, its origin will lie in a disturbance of human relationships. This may be in any area of his life—his attitude to parents, wife, girl-friend, children, employer, workmates or himself—but it will concern people rather than mere things or events. Intellectual knowledge alone is insufficient to unravel the complex strands that have woven his life. The cords are woven with emotion, not logic, so it is the emotional ties which bind him that must be examined and understood.

John, for instance (page 48), was torn between wanting to fulfil his ambition and the dawning realisation that this would entail leaving home. The prospect of leaving the people he had known and depended upon all his life was too much for him, but his interest in his chosen career did not lessen and so he remained depressed until he was able to solve his personal dilemma. In one respect it is true that he should have thought this out earlier, since it was obvious that he could not be a computer programmer unless he went to live near a computer centre, but we have already seen that his problem is an emotional rather than an intellectual or logical one.

It was precisely because he had devoted all his time and energy to intellectual advancement that his emotional development had been neglected. He needed encouragement to move in a wider circle so that he could meet more people and have the opportunity to develop satisfying personal relationships on a deeper level with some of them. He required help to understand what it was that still held him so much to home, and the as yet unformulated fears that were preventing him from embarking on a life of his own.

Most of us know the 'Monday morning' feeling and have at other times experienced a 'fit of the blues'. If a great friend unexpectedly drops in or someone phones up with good news at such a time everything immediately seems brighter. It is a very temporary condition, easily influenced by the people we meet and the things that happen around us. It is quite different from a depressive illness, which involves the whole person, and is outside the range or normal variation of mood which is experienced in a state of health and well-being.

Without treatment Alice Jones would have remained severely depressed for many months or possibly several years. A reactive depression such as John's is seldom as severe, but it may be even more protracted and certainly accounts for a great deal of waste in terms of reduced efficiency and increased unhappiness. Although it was caused by psychological rather than physical factors, it was just as much outside his control and he was equally in need of skilled treatment to help him get over it.

Unresolved spiritual issues may also give rise to depressive features. This source of conflict must always be remembered when assessing the various factors which may combine to produce a depression. Spiritual causes are deliberately mentioned only briefly, not because they are unimportant but because other people are more competent to deal with this particular aspect of the subject.

5

NORMAL AND ABNORMAL FEARS

For the first time since moving into their new bungalow, Jennifer M. was alone for the night. Her husband was attending a two-day conference in the North and as there was nothing very interesting on television she decided to write a few letters. Suddenly there was a slight scuffle followed by a muffled but unmistakable bump in the hall just outside. With pounding heart she looked round the room, resolutely picked up a heavy ornamental paperweight and flung open the door to investigate.

Limping towards her was a grey cat with a freshly torn ear and bedraggled appearance. Jennifer laughed with relief, secured the loose window through which the stray had entered and took him off to the kitchen. Fear in such circumstances is not only inescapable, it is essential to maintain life. It is both a protective and an energising force that wakens people to danger and equips them to deal with it effectively.

Fear as a normal response makes the person sit up and take notice, it makes him more alert and watchful. At the onset of danger various glands suddenly spring into action, bringing the whole person—every part and aspect of him—into the best possible state of readiness to deal with the situation. He becomes 'tuned up' and ready for a fight with, or flight from, the cause of his fear.

The mind concentrates on the immediate situation and ignores all other claims for the time being. Blood is diverted from organs whose activity is not essential at the moment and is redirected to the lungs, brain and muscles, the heart beating most forcefully to speed it on its way. Breathing becomes quicker and deeper so that more oxygen is taken into the body and waste gases can be expelled. A person who reacts like this is operating as his Creator intended, in a perfectly co-ordinated, well-balanced and purposive way.

An alarm is normally followed by action which deals with and disposes of the threat. The aim of this action is to allay fear and so restore inner harmony. Sometimes this does not happen and an alarm evokes a paralysing rather than an energising effect. The fear which it produces is more than this particular individual can turn into positive, appropriate action and he becomes unable to deal adequately with the situation confronting him. Instead of a fight against or flight from the source of the fear, he will just 'fold up'.

A reaction like this arises when a series of environmental pressures act upon a person who is, for a variety of reasons, unable either to resist or shrug them off. These pressures come first from the parents, then from the slightly wider influence of friends and school, and later from the dictates of society which make themselves felt in many different ways.

This reaction of 'folding up' in response to stress can be brought about by means intended to produce the opposite. A susceptible child whose parents are severe and domineering will have little chance of developing his individuality and becoming self-reliant. Alternatively, if he has over-indulgent parents who protect him from the stimulus necessary for personal expansion and growth he will again be ill equipped to fend for himself. Instead of rising up and responding to stress in a purposeful way, such children retreat in dismay when their parents are not around to deal with trouble for them. Each time they are unable to manage on their own or are not allowed to try, their confidence in themselves will be further undermined.

Sometimes, instead of completely paralysing a person, fear which cannot be adequately dealt with at the time it occurs will reappear later in life whenever there is any reminder of the original situation. Had Jennifer M. not had the courage to investigate that noise in the hall she would have been pursued by fear for the rest of the night. Her fear was entirely appropriate to the circumstances, and quickly abated when she dealt with the cause. On the other hand, when a person is repeatedly afraid that there might be burglars *even though he can neither see nor hear anything to suggest their presence*, such fear is inappropriate to the actual circumstances. It is a reaction to something other than the present situation.

In such cases the unconscious factors which govern and perpetuate the fears must be tracked down. They have to be rendered conscious before they can be brought under the control of the will. A person may not know what is disturbing him but he becomes aware that something is, when he experiences the bodily effects of anxiety. His heart pounds away, there seems to be a whole cageful of butterflies where his stomach normally resides and he has perhaps a host of other symptoms which he cannot account for.

When such episodes occur at all frequently it is helpful to take note of the circumstances in which they arise. Careful examination of the events and personalities involved will eventually reveal what they have in common. In this way it is often possible to determine the nature of the underlying fear-provoking stimulus. A person can only come to terms with his anxiety when he knows what is really making him anxious.

Roger G. had just such a problem. He was dismayed to experience all the physical symptoms of severe anxiety whenever he was challenged about his faith at work. He was particularly ashamed to find himself trembling as he spoke of the reality of Christ in his own experience, in answer to the challenge of an atheist. He became disturbed and disheartened at his failure to overcome this, and whenever he prayed about it he became even more anxious which, of course, increased his distress.

He began to worry about this and thought that there was something lacking in his faith. He began to imagine that he might not even be a Christian because he became so unaccountably afraid when called upon to acknowledge his personal belief and trust in Jesus Christ. Now that was an incorrect, though very understandable, assessment of the trouble; it was a complete red herring.

It took some considerable time to help him understand that his anxiety really had nothing to do with his faith, or supposed lack of it. It was due to the *status* rather than the statements of the colleague concerned, who happened to be Roger's immediate boss. Whenever the subject of religion came up, Roger—far from being the faithless failure that he had begun to consider himself—affirmed his belief, in the presence and against the declared views of his superior.

It was because he stood his ground against his senior that he became so excessively anxious. His feeling about and attitude towards his boss at work, not faith in his Lord, needed looking into and adjusting. It was anxiety at the prospect of displeasing Authority which caused his symptoms, rather than the actual subject matter of the disputes. Daring to differ with his superior revived fears which originated in his early relationship with his father. It was this that had to be examined and understood so that persisting infantile attitudes could be exposed and encouraged to mature.

Roger's father always expected too much of him as a child, continually pointing out his faults and shortcomings but seldom noticing his achievements. Not being a naturally robust personality, the boy came to accept the opinions and wishes of his father as the only right ones and gradually ceased to have any that were truly his own. As an adult he continued to feel guilty and fearful whenever he asserted his own views, no matter what the topic, and this fear was always worse whenever anything in the situation reminded him of his father.

His symptoms of anxiety were not dispelled by his earnest prayer for courage to be a more effective witness at work *because that was not his real problem.* When the origin of his fear was unravelled it could be dealt with by the man in ways that were not possible to him when he was a boy. By dealing with the root of the fear he became free to act in the present as the adult he had become, instead of continuing to react as the child he had been.

It is not difficult to see how fear can be transferred from an earlier situation on to a current one that resembles the original in some respect, but there is not always any obvious and apparent connection. Fear is frequently displaced from its original object and attached to one that has a symbolic rather than an actual significance. Anything may become the focus of such pathological fear, but certain ones are particularly common, such as a dread of any open space or an inability to travel by tube or bus.

Some people have an irrational horror of contact with a particular animal while others have an intense dread of catching an infection, any hypothetical infection. Their lives are dominated by the elaborate precautions each must take in order to avoid the feared situation. Such phobias are a compromise solution. They are an attempt to master severe anxiety but in doing so they limit the activities and restrict the lives of the sufferers.

June B. had been married for five years and gave no sign of

emotional disorder until one summer she began making all sorts of excuses for not going out. She prevailed on various neighbours to get most of the shopping during the week and her husband went with her at week-ends, but she would go nowhere without him. It was difficult to determine exactly when, or why, the trouble began until after several interviews she disclosed that sometime during the spring her mother-in-law had moved into a flat in the next block.

Superficially they got on well together but this new arrangement was too much for June. A secret resentment and jealousy flared up whenever she saw the very close relationship her husband had with his mother. She could not admit these feelings even to herself, and so strong did they become that she wanted to run away and escape what she felt to be an intolerable humiliation. Rather than do this she developed acute anxiety whenever she tried to go out at all. She was so afraid of the primitive savagery of her emotions that she became a virtual prisoner in the very building where they were most intense.

Irrational fears are very difficult for the individual to cope with and distressing to experience. They arise from unconscious conflicts which often have only a slender connection with the situation that is consciously feared. To feel afraid and not know of what you are afraid is intolerable, so when fear of the unknown rears its head, the mind immediately seeks an object for the fear. Why one situation rather than another is chosen for this will depend on the personal circumstances and background of the particular individual.

As Lord Peter Wimsey is made to remark, 'But you can't keep your feelings out of the case. It's no use saying vaguely that sex is at the bottom of all these phenomena—that's about as helpful as saying that human nature is at the bottom of them. Sex isn't a separate thing fuctioning away all by itself. It's usually found attached to a person of some sort.'[1]

The particular hallmark of pathological fear is that it is emotionally determined. It arises from within the person who is threatened by his own more or less precarious adjustment rather than by danger from the actions of other people or outside events. In certain circumstances the feeling part of his mind takes precedence over his rational judgment and his will, rather than working in harmony with them as it does in full health.

It is quite useless to tell people suffering in this way that there is 'nothing to be afraid of', because to them there certainly is. Although others can see nothing frightening in the situation, to them it is truly terrifying. This is not the rational fear of a definite, known situation, external to the person and observable by others; it arises from within himself because of his past experiences. These are his misfortune and not his fault, as is assumed by those who tell him to 'pull himself together'.

This type of fear is based on wrong interpretations and misconceptions. Although speedy removal of it would make life more comfortable for the moment, it would not correct the faulty attitude on which it is based. Such fears are like the

[1] Dorothy L. Sayers, *Gaudy Night* (Four Square).

tip of an iceberg, the only obvious evidence of a much more widespread hazard lurking underneath. They are a warning beacon which must not be ignored, a beacon calling attention to a hidden danger which is upsetting the emotional adjustment of the individual.

The individual should pray for understanding of his disability, as well as for relief from it. Too often prayer is concentrated on seeking relief from disabling fear, rather than on strength and courage to find out what he *really* fears. Only when that is known can it be faced and dealt with.

One sign may herald an approaching storm and when it is discerned the prudent take appropriate action. A restless, uneasy, dissatisfied, fearful view of life may be due to the unrest of unbelief, but it may equally be the result of unconscious emotional conflict. Both are negative conditions and the symptoms exist to draw attention to the need for appropriate action.

Although the two conditions may, and often do, co-exist each must be dealt with separately and positively. Unbelief needs to be transformed into a positive faith in God, and unconscious problems need to be made conscious.

The processes whereby these two results are achieved are quite separate and distinct. Solving unconscious conflicts certainly does not bring spiritual salvation and being spiritually transformed, renewed by faith, will not result in the automatic resolution of emotional problems. Indeed, either event alone may well bring the need for the other into greater prominence. Where this is so, it must be given full consideration or the person will remain incomplete. Only by attending to both spiritual and emotional factors will a person grow to the full extent of which he is potentially capable.

The liberation which comes when previously unconscious attitudes are brought under conscious scrutiny and control cannot take the place of divine forgiveness and acceptance. The transformation from a state of unbelief to the possession of a vital, living faith does not bring relief from unconscious problems—on the contrary, it may highlight them.

Salvation and sanity must never be confused. There is a separate and distinct pathway to each goal. Many people become discouraged because they unthinkingly expect to solve emotional problems by spiritual exercises, endeavouring to use their faith as a short cut to emotional maturity. They fail to realise that, used in this way, it becomes a hindrance rather than a help.

The assumption that a Christian should be exempt from the type of irrational and disabling fear that afflicted June B. (and many like her), increased her distress. A false and unnecessary feeling of guilt is added to already fear-laden people when they are admonished to remember that 'perfect love casts out fear', the implication being of course, that if they loved God more they would fear whatever they do fear so much less. Battering a person with isolated texts of this sort is equivalent to a hasty and intemperate slap on the face.

The object of pathological fear, as we have already seen, is not the real source of disquiet. The symptom itself will never be influenced by direct frontal attack, it will only be affected by a modification of the underlying attitudes, both conscious and unconscious.

After reading a magazine article of mine, a woman wrote to say, 'I often feel that I would be far happier if I were not a Christian and then I would not have to go to church at all. It is very hard to be a "keen Christian" when one is like this.' She was putting the cart before the horse, the outward activity of a Christian before the personal relationship with Christ from which it flows.

The problem itself was not as important as the way she faced it. Weighed down by anticipation of the fear she would experience when called upon to go out, she allowed this to rob her of the power to do anything at all. She was ashamed of her fear and in trying to hide it she made herself worse. Unwilling to confide in anyone she was unable to make friends, and became isolated and despondent. She could not be free to enjoy the company of others until she allowed them to see her as she really was, without the intolerable strain of keeping up appearances.

It needs a conscious effort to stop borrowing trouble. Faith and anticipated fear are mutually exclusive. To review the expected hurdles of each current day and deliberately give them over to God is a matter of the will. Nothing is gained by worrying all Monday about the meeting one ought to attend on Tuesday. Problems and fears cannot be avoided and should not be denied but they must not be allowed to take the central place. That belongs to God alone.

Sometimes when blind, unreasoning panic threatens to overwhelm, there is nothing that can be done *at that moment* but cling to the knowledge that nothing and no one can separate a Christian from the love of Christ. The Apostle Paul, having survived many trials and perplexities, triumphantly wrote: 'I have become absolutely convinced that neither death nor life, neither messenger of Heaven nor monarch of earth, *neither what happens today nor what may happen tomorrow*, neither a power from on high nor a power from below, nor anything else in God's whole world has any power to separate us from the love of God in Christ Jesus our Lord!' (Rom. 8. 38, 39, J. B. Phillips, *author's italics*).

A deep-rooted and disabling fear is likely to need psychiatric treatment, often over a considerable time, before it abates. The underlying causes gradually become conscious as treatment proceeds, but medical measures alone are not sufficient. The fundamental fears of mankind which all must face can only be met and mastered by acceptance of the gospel.

The great problem of so many people today is the horrifying meaninglessness of life itself. Lacking family ties and local loyalties they are appalled by their own isolation and insignificance. Increasing numbers of people can see no point or purpose in living at all. Some just drift aimlessly, others try to drown their questions in drink, dampen their insistence with drugs or silence them for ever in suicide.

Only the incredible fact of the incarnation of Jesus Christ can meet this great need. God came into the world as a human being in the person of Jesus Christ and experienced at first hand all the difficulties, temptations and disappointments that life affords. He knows what it is to be lonely and misunderstood, to be tired and hungry; to weep with the mingled longing and disappointment that is frustration; to sweat and seek relief in sleep. He knows what it is like to be forsaken by friends who could not grasp what was troubling Him.

He could endure this only because His mind and will and heart were totally given over to fulfilling the Divine purpose for His life. His goal was always to serve the Father, not please Himself. Because He finished His task we are not left to flounder alone but can have the living, enduring presence of Jesus Christ in every situation. To serve and follow Him gives meaning and purpose to an otherwise incomprehensible existence.

For other people the greatest problem is death, not life. They are haunted by a gnawing fear of nothingness, the terrible prospect of being snuffed out for ever. They are troubled by the thought of not being, and the only answer to this universal fear is the gospel of the resurrection.

Christianity teaches the survival of personality. We go on being recognisably ourselves after death, yet not as we are now. Because Christ rose from the dead, those who believe in Him will also. Other religions give meaning to death, but Jesus Christ came to give life, and to give it more abundantly.

For yet others the main problem of life is a pervading sense of guilt which they can never dispel. Guilt and fear are extremely common symptoms in psychiatric practice and it is important to ascertain whether or not there is an external, objective reason for them. If there is not and it is established that they arise from internal, subjective sources, then the unconscious conflict giving rise to them must be dealt with. The psychiatric aspect of guilt will be dealt with in the next chapter, but a guilty fear that arises from a sense of breaking the moral law of God can be met only by the atonement of Jesus Christ on the cross.

There is a perfectly normal and healthy fear that is designed to lead us to God. Fear is normal and purposive, but some fears are inappropriate to the circumstances. These have to be dealt with by indirect methods. Christ does not promise automatic deliverance *from* fear whatever its source, but He does offer strength and wisdom to *deal with the cause*.

6

MORAL AND PATHOLOGICAL GUILT

To fill in the time while waiting for his wife to emerge from the hairdressers, George T. whistled to himself as he polished the car. A few seconds elapsed before the deep voice penetrated his dreams. 'And just what do you think you're doing?' it asked. He lifted an eyebrow in mild surprise, looked slowly but uncomprehendingly up at his questioner and drawled, 'Polishing the car.'

The traffic warden silently pointed up to the red-circled 'No Waiting' notice right beside him, and down at the continuous yellow lines on the road. At that moment Karen T. appeared in the shop doorway, resplendent and radiant. The warden, intercepting the look in her husband's eye, watched appreciatively as she walked over to them, and grinned understandingly. He wished them luck, reminded George to use the proper car park next time, and proceeded on his beat with lighter steps.

George caused no obstruction and intended no harm. His accidental oversight of the 'No Waiting' order was entirely inadvertent and no moral guilt can be attached to such an insignificant and minor infringement of the regulations. Legally, of course, ignorance of the law does not prevent one from being judged guilty when one is proved to have disobeyed it, but no sensible person would have taken this particular matter any further.

Anyone who violates an accepted standard, be it legal, moral or theological, is guilty in that respect, regardless of whether or not he also 'feels guilty' at having done so.

It is important to realise that genuine guilt is not limited to legal guilt. A person is morally guilty if he fails to live up to his own accepted and realistically based principles of life, regardless of whether or not those principles have the sanction of law to enforce them. Conversely, a person who disobeys a particular law may not regard this as a moral, even though he knows and accepts that it is a legal, infringement of the law.

For our purposes it is sufficient to define moral guilt as a healthy sense of shame felt by a reasonably mature person over an actual wrong done. It must be carefully distinguished from pathological guilt, which is an unrealistic, inner, subjective sense of having done wrong. Pathological guilt is an emotionally determined attitude about oneself based on feeling without fact, or with insufficient fact to back it up. An over-anxious, insecure but innocent child may blush and appear uncomfortable when the teacher looks at the class after announcing that there is a shilling missing from the dinner money.

People are usually dismayed, and not infrequently annoyed, when fined for a motoring offence. They do not necessarily feel guilty about their offence although there can be no shadow of doubt that they are guilty in fact and in law. Even when they have taken a deliberate risk and clearly knew that they were doing wrong, they still do not necessarily feel guilty. The varying reactions of different people will depend upon their different social training and circumstances.

Vera M. was impatient to become a competent driver in as short a time as possible. In order to achieve this she behaved in a manner that would have been utterly impossible for someone of another temperament and from another background. Although she had only a provisional licence and there was no qualified person to accompany her, she decided to go out and practise by herself one fine summer evening.

Not many yards from home she stalled the car—right in the middle of the road. To her horror she saw a policeman approaching. Suddenly she remembered that her Road Fund Licence was not displayed, as it should be, on the windscreen and her 'L' plates were all too visible on the back seat. In her hurry to get out and get going she had left the licence on the hall table and had not stopped to hide the hated 'L' plates. Despite the fact that she was deliberately committing at least three illegalities there was no trace of guilt amongst her varied emotions.

Anxious that the policeman should not notice any of her transgressions Vera engaged him in cheery conversation as soon as he drew near. She pulled quickly at the self-starter and while trying to get the engine going again made a joke about her poor performance. With a completely disarming smile she said, 'Isn't it amazing what the mere sight of a policeman can do to one?' He laughed and suggested that she might get on better if she put the choke in. Thankfully she did so, and drove off to enjoy the rest of the evening feeling very pleased with herself. Although she had undoubtedly done wrong, and knew it, she felt no guilt.

By contrast some legally and morally innocent people feel acutely uncomfortable at the mere sight of a policeman. There is no objective ground for this reaction, they have done nothing wrong and their guilty feelings are inappropriate to the actual here-and-now situation. This being so, one must look else-where for the cause of their discomfort and it is readily found in that symbol of authority, the policeman's uniform.

Before going further into the question of pathological guilt we must briefly consider the Christian answer to the problem of guilt in general. Anyone who is conscious that there is some-thing wrong between God and himself must acknowledge this. The state of sin, which is rebellion against and consequent alienation from God, can only be dealt with in His appointed way. While the rebellion continues, the relationship between that man and God is broken *but it can be restored*.

When sin is acknowledged and forgiveness sought, the barrier falls away and the individual is given new life, new hope and a new sense of purpose. This new life does not mean that the individual will never do wrong again, nor that he will never want to do wrong. What it does do is to give a new awareness of what is right and what is wrong in the sight of God. It also gives the person a new strength to admit when he is wrong, and new power to overcome the tendency to sin.

No one need continue to feel guilty before God unless he chooses to. In the New Testament revelation of God there is nothing that cannot be forgiven except the refusal to accept forgiveness. When God forgives, He also forgets and blots out the record of what has been wrong. When sin is acknowledged forgiveness is freely given. If guilty feelings persist unabated after such acknowledgement it can only be because there is another aspect to the matter which makes it a fundamentally different situation. Being a different situation it calls for a different answer. It is no longer a question of sin, but of sickness.

Guilt has to do with fear of punishment. When there can be nothing to fear because sin has been confessed and forgiven, any persistent feelings of guilt are unjustified by the facts of the situation. They are due to attitudes carried over from other occasions and do not really belong in the present. This explains why some innocent people feel guilty at the mere sight of a policeman.

Guilt of this sort is basically an immature emotion. It is what a child feels when he realises that he has desires and impulses which call for actions contrary to the standards and wishes imposed on him by others. Ideally, some workable solution to this inevitable conflict of civilisation is achieved during childhood and adolescence, but in practice varying aspects of it remain unresolved.

Very early in life standards of good and bad behaviour are

taken over by the child from the standards he observes in his parents. It is not so much on what they say as on what they are and how they act that his observations are based. He learns to repeat the things which please them and to avoid as far as possible the things which excite their displeasure. What is good to them becomes good and desirable to him, and what is sensed to be bad in their estimation becomes his bad also.

Although originating from the parents, these standards of good and bad become part of the child and the feelings associated with them can then be aroused when he is alone. Soon he will have to start the long task of emancipating himself from the second-hand code of conduct taken over wholesale from his parents, and forming standards that are truly his own.

As he grows older and mixes with a wider circle of companions, he will discover that what is bad in one family is neutral or even good in another. He will start testing out, in various ways, the standards he has hitherto accepted as absolute and he will gradually form ones that are truly part of his own personality. These will still conflict with his desires and impulses at times, but as such standards are an integral part of himself rather than a foreign importation, they will not make him react with blind rage or induce unrealistic guilt.

In our society it is the aggressive and sexual drives which are most frequently and consistently checked, and so it is the emerging manifestations of these which frequently underlie pathological guilt. When a child realises that giving expression to certain of his impulses will displease his parents, he is in a dilemma. To act upon those impulses will surely bring disapproval, if not punishment, so he will feel rejected and un-loved if he yields to them, but he cannot totally deny that he has such instinctual drives. If he manages to express them in a controlled and acceptable manner he will have learnt a valuable social lesson. If for any reason he is unable to find such a solution he will retreat from the difficulty. He will push the impulse, and all feelings connected with it, out of conscious awareness.

We have already seen (chapter two) how these impulses do not just cease to exist, but operate as it were underground. Being underground, they are excluded from the continuous development that occurs in the rest of the personality, and so they retain their infantile characteristics.

If the early display of potent emotion is punished or criti-cised, a sensitive child is likely to feel that the emotion itself is wrong, not just the manner in which it was displayed. Chil-dren all too easily transfer condemnation of certain ways of displaying emotion on to the actual basic emotion itself. They will then attempt to deny that emotion any expression, instead of allowing it to remain morally neutral and trying to express it in a more acceptable manner.

Frequent, harsh punishment of temper, for instance, makes children regard any display of anger, in any situation, as wrong or dangerous. When this happens an important source of energy will be lost from their adult lives. They will not only be afraid of anger in themselves but are likely to be intolerant and excessively afraid of it in others. We usually dislike in others what we cannot accept in ourselves. This is a common source of trouble wherever people live or work closely together—the pot calling the kettle black.

A person who has repressed his aggressive drive will lack the normal amount of self-assertion necessary to get on in life. He will also suffer some degree of guilt and anxiety whenever he does assert himself. He will be torn between the impulse of assertion and the need to protect himself from feeling guilty when he gives way to it, an attitude that has been implanted by his earlier training. In just the same manner, as we saw in chapter three, a child can be made to feel guilty about his sexuality.

Children who approach puberty without a secure, positive attitude towards their sexual role are at a tremendous disadvantage. Sometimes they react against their feelings of inferiority, and the accompanying dependence, by developing an assumed over-rigid independence. They may become over-ambitious and tend to drive themselves too hard. They have a compulsion to work and get ahead, to excel in whatever they do, but however much they excel it does not really bring them satisfaction.

They lack a sense of fulfilment because they are acting under constraint, not from free adult choice. Because inwardly they feel so inferior and inadequate they strive to be without fault, which is an unobtainable condition.

They are vulnerable to the slightest hint of criticism, constantly in danger of being found out and having their inner weakness exposed. The more this danger threatens them, the more it increases their struggle to get ahead of other people,

F

and try to stay there. They have a guilty secret which must not be exposed.

People whose independence is a disguise and a compensation for persistent, unconscious dependence find it hard to accept spontaneous gestures of goodwill. They are under inner compulsion to try and make their own way without the help they secretly crave. They may have difficulty not only in accepting from others but also in genuinely giving to them. This makes any real reciprocal relationship impossible. It creates particular problems when dealing with members of the opposite sex.

A mature relationship between the sexes is possible only when men and women meet each other on a complementary basis rather than on one of attempted equivalence. It requires the desire and ability to both give and receive freely, a willing exchange between people of equal status. This cannot be achieved when one of them has a haunting sense of guilt about himself.

Guilt is to the psyche what pain is to the body, an indicator that something, somewhere, is wrong. Sometimes pain in the shoulder originates not from the joint or muscle in that region but from something irritating the diaphragm, which is the partition between the abdomen and chest. This curious state of affairs exists because of anatomical nerve pathways laid down during development. Similarly, because of the way the personality has developed, psychic pain in the form of guilt may be felt in one area of life when it really stems from a quite different source.

Many psychiatric symptoms seem absurd because the feeling

of guilt has been isolated from its origin and attached to another act or situation. They seem incomprehensible precisely because the underlying guilt is out of its true context, which may itself be unconscious.

Pathological guilt may be most in evidence where it is least appropriate. As Jung says, 'When we dare not acknowledge some great sin we deplore some small sin with greater emphasis.' Excessive concern over quite minor matters frequently occurs as a way of unconsciously diverting attention from something of much greater significance. The conscious mind is preoccupied with guilty feelings about a relative trifle because hidden in the unconscious are memories which are intolerable for the person to recall. The feeling remains but is diverted on to another topic.

Guilt may be displaced from one situation on to another in the same way that anxiety frequently is. This was discussed in the last chapter, and shown particularly in the case of June B. In fact, although anxiety, fear and worry cause much unhappiness they do not become deposited in the unconscious unless there was also some feeling of guilt in the original situation. Anyone with an abnormal dread of cats or cows, or anything else, may have been badly frightened by one of these creatures but physical fear alone, however intense, will not by itself produce a lasting phobia.

For this to happen there must have been some shame in the original episode, shame such as a child feels when he fails to behave in the way that is required of him. Perhaps he cried and was told not to be a baby, or ran away and was teased for being a coward. When this happens children are ashamed of their failure to live up to the standards their parents expect, and as adults they continue to feel guilty whenever they find themselves in a situation which has something in common with the original episode.

It is not uncommon for people to have a fear of dirt to such an extent that their life is disrupted by a compulsion continually to wash their hands. The contamination of which they are afraid is, however, an inner, psychological one rather than an outer, physical reality. It is an expression of guilt about something done or thought.

Sometimes guilt is the product, rather than the cause, of a severe mental illness. We saw in chapter four how an overwhelming sense of guilt may be the most conspicuous evidence of a depression. It also occurs in other illnesses and may appear in an even more startling and unusual form. Peter J., for instance, was an intelligent boy who went on to study science at University. In his second year there he began to read a great deal about astronomy and became absorbed in trying to discover the ultimate source of life and the system that controls it.

He spent more and more time reading and speculating on his own, gradually dropping out of other activities. He found it increasingly difficult to talk with other people and began to suspect that he was being laughed at in College. He developed an excessive concern with right and wrong, about which he had decidedly unusual and vehement ideas. He suffered a great deal of mental torment when he had not done something which he regarded as essential, and he felt guilty about thoughts and actions which no one else would have considered to be the least wrong or harmful.

As time went on he became suspicious of everyone, including his family, and he refused to eat because he thought that he was being poisoned. His illness had upset his judgment and his ability to think clearly. It was the illness as a whole which had to be treated, not just his preoccupation with excessive guilt. After treatment, when he was able to think and evaluate clearly again, this morbid preoccupation disappeared.

A different problem was presented by Anita B., who also turned against eating. She continued to do well at work and to feel well in herself but she would not eat. Once rather plump, she decided to diet and did it so drastically that in her late teens she was little more than a skeleton and still she would not eat. She would talk to people about any subject other than her own feelings and fears. She felt very threatened by any emotional arousal. So she kept all her feelings locked up inside herself; she was even unaware that they existed.

Anita could not discuss her problems rationally until she recognised they existed. It was her total loss of appetite that showed she had problems. She needed help before she could acknowledge her emotional difficulties and then she had to be assisted to face rather than evade them. She had reason to feel guilty about certain things but at first she did not do so, because they were too painful for her to admit even to herself.

In this case it was the task of the psychiatrist to bring the unacknowledged guilt out into the open, and to discuss how

Anita might deal with the matter that had provoked it. But he could not go further. Whether she actually did anything as a result of their discussions was something she alone could decide.

Peter had a mental illness which needed medical and psychological treatment. Like everybody else he also had spiritual needs but these were not prominent during his treatment. Anita had both psychological and moral problems which needed to be disentangled. Each of these then had to be dealt with separately in their own right.

In any battle we need to know the position of the enemy so that he can be enticed out of hiding and confronted openly. Only when an enemy is recognised as an enemy will his habits be studied so that his position can be tracked down. In practical terms the things of which we are ashamed, and which we therefore try to keep hidden, are emotions which persist as infantile, uncontrollable reactions.

Our adult, informed and educated selves decry those up-surges of jealousy, rage, sexuality and so on that occur with awkward persistence, but it does not help just to shut the door on them. It is more constructive to regard immature emotional reactions as noisy, troublesome children who need adult guidance and help in order to develop beyond that stage. It certainly does not help to adopt stern, punitive measures in a vain attempt to keep them out of sight. Out of sight so often means into trouble.

Much unnecessary suffering and unhappiness occurs because of our tendency to deny things of which we feel guilty. We all have thoughts and habits which we would prefer to be without, but we cannot get rid of them unless we first acknowledge that they exist. As long as they remain unrecognised, as long as we try to keep them at bay, they will continue to strike us in unexpected places like guerilla fighters in the jungle. We cannot overcome evil with good until the presence of evil has been acknowledged.

Guilt makes us want to shut things away, to push them out of our lives. Growth occurs when we accept those things which disturb us, in order that we may encourage them to develop into something better. This means recognising pathological guilt so that immature reactions may develop into mature emotions. It also calls for the confession of genuine moral guilt so that a right relationship with God and man may be achieved.

7

HIDING FROM ONESELF

As an established clerk of many years' standing in the Civil Service, David G. knew he would never be made redundant, although this had happened to several of his friends in industry. He was of average efficiency, always punctual, and plodded slowly through his allotted work. He had had no sick leave for eleven years but lately he had begun to worry about his health. He feared he might be going mad.

Words and phrases kept reverberating round his mind against his will. On the way to work in the morning it was usually the last thing he heard on the radio news. He would repeat this over and over again to himself until he reached the office and something else took its place. Fragments of conversation went round and round in his head, interfering with his concentration. He could not remember exactly when the trouble began; for some weeks it had been getting worse and now he was really afraid of losing his reason.

David had never married but lived at home with his parents, who were in good health. The atmosphere was a relaxed and pleasant one, he had no financial or other worries and spent most of his spare time in the greenhouse, growing rare orchids. He enjoyed an occasional visit to the pictures and sometimes dropped in at the local for an hour or two, but most of his time was spent between home and work, a quiet, unruffled life that satisfied him.

It remained unruffled on the surface but he was due for promotion. Although this entailed very little extra responsibility it was sufficient to upset him. When his fears about the impending promotion were understood they had to be brought out into the open so that he was fully conscious of them. After discussing the position and making suitable arrangements through an understanding personnel officer, his symptoms disappeared.

Many people say, 'It's just nerves, isn't it, Doctor—I'm not going mad, am I?' If their illness, whatever it is called, interferes with their lives sufficiently they will agree to go into hospital for treatment but recoil in horror when the area psychiatric hospital is named. It is the old story of 'give a dog a bad name'.

Most such hospitals in Britain were built fifty or more years ago when less was known about this type of illness and very little treatment was available. The attendants were often keepers, not nurses, who took over their job without any training. The large, barrack-like buildings had little cheer for their inmates, a considerable number of whom stayed there many years and sometimes for the rest of their lives. Today we use the same buildings but everything else has changed.

High railings, locked gates and padded cells are out; effective forms of treatment, more varied occupation and greater personal freedom are in. It is far better for someone with 'nerves' to go to a hospital where they can participate actively in the business of getting well, rather than to a general hospital where there are no facilities for them to do anything except lie in bed and brood.

People with mental and emotional disturbances live at least partly in a world of their own. They have never fully come to grips with the world of reality. There is a saying that 'Neurotics build castles in the air, psychotics go and live in them, and psychiatrists collect the rent from both.' A neurotic person to some extent realises the difference between fact and phantasy but a person who is psychotic can no longer make the distinction. His own peculiar world is 'real' to him and our real world is not.

Freud made a clear distinction between these two states when he said, 'Neurosis does not deny the existence of reality, it merely tries to ignore it; psychosis denies it and tries to substitute something else for it.' An intelligent patient with a severe emotional handicap realised this when she wrote to supplement the account given at her first interview. She said, 'Whenever it was possible I sought refuge in my own private world. The fact is that I have found so much peace and contentment in my private world that I find there are occasions when I have to force myself to realise that it is not the other one that is unreal.'

Retaining the ability to distinguish between the two worlds

does not mean that a person is less severely disabled. Although 'going mad' is always thought to be so much worse than 'having nerves', a psychosis (madness) of sudden, severe onset is far more likely to respond to treatment than is a person who has always been 'a martyr to nerves'. It is not the type of disability, but the degree and extent of it, which determines how a person copes with the crises he encounters.

Names are quite properly used to classify subjects, but sometimes they are unconsciously misused in order to obscure evade an issue. Many people say, somewhat complacently, 'It's my nerves,' as though this adequately explains all their difficulties. Merely giving a name to their trouble does not increase their understanding of themselves, or help them to master their state. They need to probe further, to find out what is behind the disturbance of normal function which has become manifest as 'nerves'.

Other people have the mistaken notion that in some way it is a betrayal of faith to have any such thing as 'nerves'. They therefore look for a different explanation of any symptoms they develop. When symptoms interfere with Christian activities some people tend to say immediately that it is 'an attack of the devil'.

This is usually a misleading and inadequate explanation. It is misleading, not because there is no such being as the devil, but because it encourages the attitude, 'Fight it off', rather than 'Let's see what this is all about.' It is inadequate, not because it is not true but because it does not question the reason for the symptoms. It jumps to a conclusion and blocks all further enquiry, including enquiry which is designed to lead to better all-round adjustment.

When nervous reactions are said, without adequate foundation, to be of satanic origin it is an example of the universal tendency to attribute unwelcome inner experiences to external agencies. It is always easier to acknowledge that one has difficulties if they can be assigned an origin outside oneself, for this enables the individual to avoid personal responsibility for the matter. By externalising and spiritualising what is primarily an inner, emotional problem attention is diverted from the turmoil within. But this inner turmoil cannot be allayed until its presence is recognised.

Many people find any mention of the devil either ridiculous or abhorrent. This is because they think only of that caricature so frequently to be seen dangling in car windows, a prancing demon in coloured tights with horns and a forked tail; or else they fear that it heralds a return to the primitive and superstitious thought of earlier ages. The biblical concept is neither of these. It is of the very personification of the principle of evil engaged in spiritual warfare directed against the person and purposes of God.

All imperfection and all breakdown in natural order are the result of an evil influence in the world which scripture calls the devil. This is certainly the ultimate cause of illness, but we must beware of naïvely assuming that the devil is the agent *immediately* responsible for any particular illness. Such an assumption deflects attention from actions of our own which we ought to alter.

Bob S., maintenance man for the headquarters of a commercial enterprise, was always busy. Continually on the go, he frequently took on jobs that were really outside his brief. Occasionally he undertook commissions 'off the record' for members of the staff, and consequently he was in great demand. After work he spent a lot of time at the Social Club where he was a member of the darts team; instructor for the Do It Yourself section; chairman of the Social Services Committee, and self-appointed Ombudsman for the entire staff. Not surprisingly, his wife hardly ever saw him, he was almost a stranger to their three children, and the family was in danger of breaking up.

Mike W., electrician in the same office block, seldom stayed late and rarely went to the Social Club but his wife also saw very little of him. They were keen supporters of the small Mission Church in the centre of the town. With choir practice, men's club, magazine distribution and sundry other commitments his spare time was fully occupied. In theory he and his wife took it in turns to go to the mid-week fellowship but Mike often had a deacons' meeting following it, or some urgent visiting to do and so he was usually the one to go.

Once a week he did try to get home in time for his wife to go to the women's meeting but other nights he frequently did not get in for his evening meal until after ten o'clock. Now some of the older youths were urging him to take them for football on Saturday afternoon. He did not like to disappoint them so he decided to stay up even later on a couple of other evenings to prepare for his Bible Class. He denied feeling tired but began to be forgetful and to look ill.

When he developed a series of painful boils, he attributed this to the devil throwing a spanner in the work. He completely overlooked the fact that his low resistance to infection was the natural outcome of poor nutrition and persistent fatigue.

No one is exempt from the natural laws governing the universe. Whenever anyone breaks those laws he will inevitably be less efficient and less fit for the service of his God. Paul appeals to the Roman Christians 'to present your bodies as a living sacrifice, holy and acceptable to God, which is your spiritual worship' (Rom. 12. 1 RSV). No heathen would dare to offer a maimed or weak beast as a sacrificial offering to his dead gods, yet we sometimes deliberately neglect our bodies, and minds, so that we present them half-dead before the Living God.

It is an insult to God, as well as a disservice to the Church and oneself, to squander the gift of health. Running about night after night on Church affairs, sitting up late at committees and organising meetings leaves some people no time for necessary relaxation and recreation. The ceaseless over-activity which leads to such an impoverished state calls for examination of the motives behind it. Sometimes the person is running away from himself. All this work is undertaken in the name of 'service' but closer inspection may reveal that the impetus really comes from the necessity to hide from himself.

Rather than being an admirable, sacrificial pursuit for no personal gain such behaviour may be the outcome of an unrecognised personality problem. When this is so it will render the person less useful and effective, less happy in himself, than he might be. He needs to pause and face his own basic difficulties, instead of continuing to evade them in perpetual religious activity.

Constant preoccupation with, and over-involvement in, the affairs of other people is often a cover for personal difficulties. The individual who is dissatisfied in his relationships at home will seek to escape from a painful awareness of this, and at the same time to provide a substitute satisfaction, by multiplying his commitments outside the family orbit. This soon becomes a vicious circle.

The more he is away from home the more likely the family are to adjust to his absences. He will be less indispensable at home and so will obtain even less satisfaction there. The result of this is a correspondingly greater internal pressure driving him on to engage in still more outside activities. He will go wherever there is a need which he can fill, and which will in turn bring him some fulfilment.

When difficulties in inter-personal relationships occur they are seldom confined to one area of life. If the hidden reason for taking on extra activities is to evade tension at home, it is inevitable that the work which is undertaken, and the unsatisfactory home life for which it compensates, are both bound to suffer. They will suffer because the tension will increase unless the source of it is dealt with. For the sake of the work, the family, and the individual concerned, personality problems of this nature must be reckoned with. If they go unrecognised, dissatisfaction at home will result in trouble at the office, the club, the Church, and wherever else that individual comes into close contact with other people.

When a person has difficulty in getting on reasonably with others at work or at home, he is unlikely to find it automatically easier within the Church. There is tremendous need for greater realism on this point. Too often it is assumed that just because people have this one thing in common they will therefore be able to work well together and that personality factors can be consequently discounted. On the contrary, they should always be taken into full consideration.

A buried personality problem will result in subtle evasion of personal contact with anyone who activates the underlying conflict. This evasion may begin and continue without the person concerned realising that he is avoiding a particular individual. He will find more or less convincing 'reasons' for sending messages via a third person, or writing a note, or just letting the matter slide; anything rather than allow a personal meeting.

For example, anyone who repeatedly finds himself 'too busy' to cross the corridor and discuss a joint endeavour whenever it concerns a particular colleague should stop and enquire why this is so. If he normally makes his plans by direct person to person consultation this repeated avoidance of a particular individual is significant. It means that communication is impaired between them, and this can have widespread results. It leads to misinterpretation, misquotation and inaccuracies which have little chance of being corrected or prevented as long as the situation continues. It will result in hard feelings on both sides, which flourish like weeds on waste ground.

The human mind is incredibly ingenious at finding socially acceptable explanations to justify what it wants to believe or to do. It readily provides reasons that disguise the real but unpalatable facts. In the example given, the excuse of 'too busy' is acceptable because there are many worthy reasons for being fully occupied. On the other hand it is not generally acceptable to admit openly that one does not want to meet a colleague when there is no rational, objective ground for not doing so. It is important to be as aware as possible of these small and apparently insignificant self-deceptions because they can so often lead to more serious difficulties. When one is conscious of the underlying motive one can take steps to compensate for it.

Again, this situation is not avoided just because all the people concerned are members of the same Church. Indeed, it may be more prevalent there because few would care to admit that they have an unaccountable dislike of the popular new churchwarden, deacon or elder. The dislike springs from unconscious sources and is quite irrational, which is a further reason for not admitting it exists. As has so often been said in this book, only when the presence of such an attitude is admitted can the effect of it be consciously controlled.

When unfounded antipathies arise, the subject should try to discover what particular aspect of the other person he finds so annoying. What characteristics, sayings, actions or mannerisms does he find irritating, and of whom do they remind him? He should follow up any and every association that comes to mind, however remote it may seem. Frequently he will be led back to some episode or person encountered in the past.

This association is important, and opens the way to improved communication between the people concerned. When a spontaneous reaction can be seen as evoked because of past events, rather than belonging in the present, it loses much of its sting. It also enables the individual to divest the disliked person of negative personal associations and to begin to meet him as a real person in his own right. He becomes less of a bogey figure invested with past problems and more of a contemporary who can be met on adult terms.

Freud has written a clear account of how meaningful such a chain of associations can be in his *Psychopathology of Everyday Life*.[1] The course to be taken must be that of moderation, the middle road between being completely unaware of one's blind spots, and becoming so fascinated with the peculiarities of the unconscious that one develops the morbid habit of perpetual self-scrutiny. One must endeavour to be aware of inter-personal difficulties without being unreasonably wrapped up in the study of them.

To some people it will come as quite a shock when they realise how skilled they have become at avoiding a particular person. Once the error is acknowledged the situation can be greatly improved by taking extra care to build up a better relationship through direct, warm, person-to-person exchanges.

[1] Published as a paperback by Collins (Comet Books).

A deliberate watch must be kept so that there is not a gradual sliding back into the old way of avoidance again.

Other people, when detecting a persistent unwelcome attitude in themselves towards another, will analyse it partially and say that it is jealousy, pride or some other 'deadly sin'. They say that they must 'repent', and are content to do the same again next time a similar situation occurs. Repentance is, of course, a necessary action after each manifestation of sin, but in this type of manifestation it is not enough. It will not remove the unconscious antipathies from which the attitude springs. The historical development of such attitudes must be understood so that they can be re-formed. The source of the trouble, rather than each isolated instance of its existence, must be dealt with.

We saw in chapter two that most nervous illness is the result of inner tension. It arises because of conflict within the personality, rather than directly because of difficulties that press in upon the individual from outside. It is when external events cause a clash of opinion within, and create a conflict that is more or less hidden from himself, that tension begins to build up. When there is a clash of loyalties the tension will continue to build up until an acceptable solution is found. If a satisfactory resolution of the dilemma cannot be found, symptoms of one sort or another will inevitably occur.

When this build up of emotional pressure cannot be appropriately discharged it will cause a predisposed individual to develop physical symptoms. Some families have a tendency to asthma and although emotional upset is not the only, and in some cases never the main, reason for an attack, it is likely to play some part in it. Our whole breathing apparatus is controlled by a delicately balanced nervous system and because of this the mechanism is very easily upset.

When a person has asthma that is primarily due to allergy or infection, he may well develop an attack when he comes under nervous strain even though the allergic or infective element is minimal at that time. When the usual precipitant has caused an attack to start it is likely to be made worse or to last longer if the person is also under strain. If, on the other hand, he develops an infection when he is emotionally more stable he will be less likely to succumb to an attack on that occasion.

Just as some people are asthmatic, so others are liable to suffer from gastro-intestinal trouble (ulcers, colitis and so on), skin disorders or a host of other bodily disturbances. This is their 'weak part' and so it determines where and how their bodies show that they are under more pressure than they can cope with. When a person has no such 'weak part' his symptoms will not be localised in this way. Instead, the evidence of conflict within will be the more generalised symptoms of anxiety, insomnia, headaches, irritability or depression.

Inner tension results in different symptoms in different people. The way a given person reacts to tension is determined by the interaction of many factors. Similar symptoms in different people do not mean that they are experiencing the same type of difficulty, and people who have similar conflicts are likely to show them in quite different ways.

Many people deny that their symptoms, whatever form they

take, can have any connection with their personal lives. They are reluctant even to consider the possibility because they do not like to think that they cannot cope with their own emotions. No progress can be made until the individual is willing to examine his personal relationships, and to admit the existence of difficulties when they are present.

A Christian is not someone who has, or who can possibly become, perfect overnight. He does not lose all his pathological fear, and pride, and jealousy, the moment he receives new life in Christ. Instead he is like a business that is 'Under New Management', as we sometimes see written in shop windows. The details of day to day administration are not all changed immediately, but the overall aim and policy is different from the previous one. The various changes that are required will be introduced gradually when the new owner sees that the individual is ready to make them.

Part of God's plan for each of us is that we should, with His help, overcome the attitudes that keep us immature. Psychological conflict remains psychological, whatever name we give it, but it does not make us any less children of God.

8

ACCEPTING ONESELF

Apart from his Carnaby Street gear there was nothing outstanding about Richard. He had given up trying to cope with his situation. He complained of being 'run down' and asked for a tonic, but his was a fatigue that no bottled tonic, no amount of rest and no long holiday could dispel. He was dissatisfied about many things, but chiefly because his parents had made it plain all his life that they wanted him to get a University degree.

Nothing else seemed acceptable to them, although eventually they agreed that he could go to the Technical College instead. He enjoyed it at first and was of above average ability, so the studying did not overtax him. Gradually he lost interest and became too lethargic even to bother with photography, his favourite hobby. Because he was so tired he started cutting lectures and halfway through the second term he was only going into College one or two half-days a week. The rest of the time he spent in his room, doing very little studying and nothing much else.

His parents paid all his fees and gave him a generous allowance. They had also found, furnished and paid the rent for a flat he shared with an older brother. Had Richard been free to make his own choice he would never have lived with that particular brother because they were temperamentally so different. In this, too, he felt a failure. He was tired out by trying to keep down the demands of his own creative bent, and by trying to keep up with an academic life for which he was not suited.

Emotional conflict is not, of course, the only cause of chronic tiredness but it is one of the most common. Anaemia and many other disorders can have exactly the same effect, and for each disorder there is a specific remedy. The specific remedy for fatigue caused by inner tension is to deal with the source of the conflict. It is, however, often a long and difficult road between recognising what the problem is, and being able to deal with it more adequately.

As the youngest child of a large and gifted family Richard had always been told what to do. He had not developed the normal amount of self-assertion and he had little confidence in his own opinion or judgment. He had first of all to define his problem and then decide what he himself really wanted to do in life, regardless of what his family expected him to be or do. This was not easy for him, and it took time. He had to be encouraged to make his own decisions so that gradually he learnt to rely more on himself, less on his family and other people.

First of all he had to accept himself as he was — accept and develop his own undoubted gifts even though these departed from the family tradition. This meant making an honest and frank appraisal of his personal strengths as well as his weaknesses. Because his talents were practical rather than academic they had been discounted; he was only conscious of being somewhat of a disappointment to his family. He was unable to talk to anyone about this and took refuge in daydreams. He needed to take stock of himself and begin to see himself as he actually was, not the person he dreamed of becoming nor the one he thought other people expected him to be.

It has been said by one experienced in dealing with the personal problems of others[1] that a person can only accept about himself things that he has openly and verbally admitted to another. If he cannot accept them in himself, he cannot tell anyone about them; if he cannot admit them to another person then they remain unacceptable to him.

The process of accepting oneself can be greatly helped if friends are honest in their observations, providing that they speak in a kindly way and not as an accusation. We always want to hide feelings of which we are for any reason ashamed, and when we see others struggling in the same way it is natural to want to go along with them in their attempted self-deception. It is far better to help them to be more open by being so ourselves.

When we see someone who is obviously nervous, or afraid, or depressed, it is important openly to acknowledge this and accept him *as he is*. From an early age we are trained to play

[1] Anthony Storr, *The Integrity of the Personality* (Pelican).

a destructive game of convenient social blindness, but as Christians we must learn the better way of honesty—honesty with ourselves, our neighbours and our God.

Dr B. learnt this by being a patient himself. Feeling somewhat morose the day after an operation, he tried all morning to hide this misery. After lunch a friend dropped in and it was not long before he bluntly said, 'The trouble with you doctors is that you always expect to be different from everyone else. You can't expect not to be affected by the strain of this, so don't go on pretending you're not feeling down.' That friend was right! Just by admitting how he was really feeling, instead of trying to hide it, Dr B. immediately felt better.

All morning the nurses had been colluding with him by pretending not to notice how depressed he was in spirit. The surgeon too was somewhat embarrassed and ill at ease. The medical and nursing staff had given skilled and excellent care to his physical state, but its emotional concomitant had been glossed over. That was something the surgeon could not chop out or sew up and he did not know what to do about it. The discerning friend saw how to deal with the situation as soon as he entered the room; he brought the hidden, unacceptable feelings out into the open.

Too often we are kept back from talking as freely as we need to because of a crippling fear of what the other person will think. When someone manages to instil in us sufficient confidence to relieve the worst of this crippling paralysis, we frequently find with relief that he understands far more than we ever expected. Often he will discover that this is because he has himself experienced much the same difficulties at some time in his life.

Knowledge of this at once takes some of the burden away, for to realise that the experience is not peculiar to oneself, and does not cut one off from others, is always a great encouragement. It seems particularly necessary for our generation, as it was for the Corinthians, to be reminded that 'no temptation has overtaken you that is not common to man' (1 Cor. 10. 13 RSV). When we realise and take hold of this fact it is not quite so difficult to talk to others on the basis of common experience.

Whatever the burden, whatever the fear or secret despair, one must not endeavour to bear it alone. If an attempt is made to do so, the weight and worry of it will go on increasing as long as it is regarded as a shame to be hidden. We are told to bear one another's burdens, and if we expect to do so for others we must not be too proud to allow them to do so for us on occasions.

Many people are ashamed to admit their need of human help and companionship, yet it is essential for growth and health. Certain sections of the Church seem peculiarly liable to perpetuate a tendency to neurotic withdrawal from people. This stems from a misunderstanding of the doctrine 'Christ alone is sufficient'. Some people wrongly take this to imply 'Christ ought to be sufficient alone', meaning without human aid. That is just not true. This must not be taken to suggest any limitation of the sovereign power and all-sufficiency of Christ. It is stressed in order to draw attention to the fact that

He normally works through, and not instead of, the agency of other people.

Men and women like George Muller and Gladys Aylward relied solely on God for the provision of all their needs. Whether they required food and clothing, or transport across the Yellow River for large numbers of people it was always supplied in answer to believing prayer.[1] Often the answer came in totally unexpected and unforeseen ways but however it came it was always through other human beings. Even when Elijah survived a long famine on rations brought by ravens (I Kings 17. 6) it must be noted that God directed one of His creatures to supply the need. He did not cause food to drop directly out of an empty sky. Neither will He relieve our distress if we wilfully insist on remaining isolated and alone.

As social beings we need to be continually in contact with other people. We need the stimulation of exchanging ideas and thoughts, joys and sorrows, hopes and fears, with our companions on the journey of life. It is by sharing things of common concern, especially basic emotional reactions and desires, and by having respect for the genuine differences found in others, that we develop our own individual personalities.

Just as the body will slowly die if no food is taken in, so the personality shrivels and withers away if it is not continually nourished by regular contact with other people.

Shortly after Creation God said, 'It is not good that the

[1] Alan Burgess, *The Small Woman* (Pan).

man should be alone' (Gen. 2. 18), and so a companion was immediately provided. When Christ sent his band of followers out into the surrounding districts He did not send them alone, but in pairs. They needed the presence of each other for companionship as well as for mutual protection from physical dangers. They could not adequately fulfil their great commission alone, for they needed someone with whom to share the hopes and heartaches of each day. The different contribution each could make to the other would further their common task as they went along.

We all need the opportunity of sharing our thoughts and feelings with others. Christ Himself longed for His three closest friends to remain awake during His ordeal in the garden of Gethsemene. He felt let down and terribly alone when He found them sleeping, unable to remain awake when He was so troubled. As our Lord and Master needed companionship while on earth, so do we all our days.

Often it is only as we discuss a problem with others that the issues involved become clear enough for us to see a means of solution. This discussion may well take place alone with God; frequently, however, it will need the help of trusted friends and sometimes it may require the professional help of someone skilled at unravelling the unconscious elements that cause the problem to persist. A condition of any complexity will need considerable time and repeated discussion before the way out becomes clear. Rome was not built in a day!

One of the greatest privileges that a Christian has is to 'carry everything to God in prayer'. If help is to be gained from doing so, then it must really be a full and frank disclosure of one's actual condition at the time. How can anyone talk freely to God about the things that he has not yet really admitted to himself? Most of us try to be too respectable in our private prayer life as well as in our outward, more or less conventional, social life. We need to learn again the uncompromising frankness of men like Job and Jeremiah whose prayers are quite startling to us in their completely open disclosure of inner turmoil. See, for example, Job 7 and Jeremiah 20. 7-18.

Some people are unable to make friends even when they do mix freely with others. This is usually because they never really get to know the person behind an occupational 'label'. They allow themselves to be led away from the real person by the image of the 'type' that they expect him to be. They anticipate that anyone with authority (a teacher, solicitor, or bank manager) will be unapproachable and perhaps always looking for fault. They forget that he may also have habits and interests unconnected with his work.

Rather diffidently greeting a newcomer to the church, Mrs Clarke was somewhat overawed to learn that the thin woman beside her was a Ward Sister at St Peter's. She seemed to be only about her own age too. No, she hadn't been there long; yes, she liked it very much; no, she hadn't any friends in the area yet. Her accent was from the other end of England. Mary Clarke badly wanted to invite this stranger to her home but hesitated to do so, wondering whether she could suitably entertain a person whose experience and training she assumed to be so much wider than her own.

That stranger had a comfortable bed-sitting room, though it was on the small side. The Nurses Home had swing entrance doors, a large vestibule that was usually uncomfortably empty; and long, bare corridors. Instead of lessening the institutional atmosphere the potted plants on the window-sills and elsewhere somehow contrived to make it more obvious. There was a common room with television, of course, and a reasonable kitchen for the exclusive use of the Sisters but everything about the place reminded her of work.

Dawn Price wanted to get a flat and was looking for someone to share it with, for the companionship as well as for reasons of economy. She ran her ward well and was liked by the nurses, but after work she longed to relax her vigilance and share the daily routine as an equal, not a leader. She wanted to break out of the pattern imposed by her uniform.

Several Sundays later, waiting in the porch for the heavy rain to ease a little, Dawn and Mary got talking. They discovered a common interest in books and book-binding. Before the storm was over Mary had invited Dawn to spend her next day off with her. It was not long before a warm friendship sprang up between them and Mary one day admitted how different Dawn was from her picture of a tyrannical and implacable Ward Sister.

In order to make friends one must get into effective contact with a real person, not just a stereotyped idea of one. Of course this also means being prepared to drop one's own mask in order to let others get to know the real person, with real feelings, behind it.

Sometimes this is made difficult by the individual's own inner, and usually unacknowledged, idea of the sort of person he would like to be. This sets up an ideal of how he ought to behave in order to conform to his expectations of himself. It inhibits spontaneity, which can only be restored when the person accepts himself as he actually is, rather than as he wants to be, and allows his genuine feelings some expression. He must drop his pose and become a person again.

An individual is always more effective when he learns to work along with, rather than struggling against, the forces of his own nature. These vary not only from person to person but also in any one person from time to time. Rhythmic cycles occur widely in the whole of nature: day and night; the yearly seasons observed in the prevailing weather; times of growth, harvest and dying away again. In our bodies and minds too the balance of chemical control is constantly shifting.

Even the body temperature of a healthy person is not absolutely constant. It is usually slightly higher in the evenings and lowest in the early hours of the morning (between three and six am), with the rhythm reversed in night workers. The level of sugar circulating in the blood is also lowest in the early morning and it varies within certain normal limits throughout the day. Then too there are the more obvious changes in the monthly cycle of a woman and these frequently include alterations in her mood, energy and vigour.

Many people have their own slight but distinct and perfectly normal cycle of active phases alternating with periods of comparative lethargy and disinterest. C. S. Lewis has described

111

this in his Screwtape letter on the law of Undulation.[1] He says: 'As spirits they (humans) belong to the eternal world, but as animals they inhabit time. This means that while their spirit can be directed to an eternal object, their bodies, passions and imaginations are in continual change, for to be in time means to change. Their nearest approach to constancy, therefore, is undulation — the repeated return to a level from which they repeatedly fall back, a series of troughs and peaks. If you had watched . . . carefully you would have seen this undulation in every department of his life — his interest in his work, his affection for his friends, his physical appetites, all go up and down. As long as he lives on earth periods of emotional and bodily richness and liveliness will alternate with periods of numbness and poverty.'

When faced with difficulties some people tend to withdraw into themselves and away from their fellows, rather as a tortoise will retire into its shell if it is at all roughly handled. Others who are by temperament more outgoing find it easier to pour out their problems to whoever is nearest, without pausing to reflect at all. They are like puppies, always jumping up at anyone within reach.

The puppy behaviour, like that of the tortoise, prevents contact with others. In this case it is the other person who withdraws, in self-defence, from the emotional onslaught. Both these reactions need to be adjusted so that they do not lead to a break in personal relationships. No tortoise can become a puppy, or vice versa, but each can endeavour to modify their

[1] C. S. Lewis, *The Screwtape Letters* (Fontana).

reactions so that they encourage, rather than repel, other people.

Success in personal relationships does not lie in an excess of one reaction or the other, but in a right balance between the two. As usual when dealing with extremes of any sort, what is needed is the middle way between being too fearful to share anything with anyone at all, and an indiscriminate sharing of everything with everybody.

Those who are by nature contemplative often feel ashamed when they see how men of action respond to crises. Peter was able to sleep soundly in prison the night before his trial, even though chained between two strong, well-trained soldiers. He was an explosive man who dealt with his problems by externalising them. He discharged his feelings in quick, impulsive reactions that were more likely to cause trouble by their effect on others than within himself.

Coming to terms with ourselves means accepting the limitations as well as the exciting possibilities of our own particular nature. It is the task of each individual to develop his gifts to the full, without in the process looking over his shoulder at someone else and wishing that he had been made like that person instead of as he is. It is not, however, always easy to know when we are essentially without a certain ability, and when we have in fact got the capacity but have not yet succeeded in getting it to develop.

The first state must be accepted as final but it is even more imperative to recognise the second, in order to remedy it. Often it is not until a person mixes with others who are using the very ability that lies dormant in himself that he becomes aware of his undeveloped potential. When he does become dimly aware of it he can either take the opportunity to expand, or turn away and retreat from the possibility.

Anyone who grasps and uses the opportunity to widen his horizons will become a more complete person, while those who turn their backs on it will remain limited in outlook and personality. The way to achieve wholeness is by taking every opportunity for a fuller, richer, more satisfying and stimulating life in every sphere of being.

9

A CARING COMMUNITY

Nearly twenty and never having needed a doctor before, Elizabeth G. did not know whose advice to take. Now in her second year at Bible College, she had been feeling unwell for a couple of weeks. Twice she nearly fainted in lectures and was then admitted to hospital for investigation. The doctors in charge thought that her trouble was largely psychological and when all the tests proved normal they were sure. When they suggested she should be transferred to a psychiatric hospital for further observation, the Principal of her College told her he would not have her back if she went to that type of hospital.

He told her that it would be a denial of her Christian faith to go—an untenable statement which this book has endeavoured to disprove.

The assumption that mental illness and emotional disorder are marks of spiritual disgrace cannot be too strongly refuted. They are no more disgraceful than a broken leg! There is no place in the 'pull yourself together' brigade for any thinking Christian.

One person in every ten people resident in the United Kingdom will require psychiatric treatment at some time in his life. For one in fifteen this will be in a mental hospital (one in eight of those over forty). In terms of families, one family in five will have one member who suffers from a disabling mental illness. This is due to more frequent recognition rather than to any increase in the amount of such illness this century. As public awareness increases, and more effective means of treatment are devised, more provision for treatment has to be made available.

No single facet of life protects a person from becoming mentally ill. No immunity is given by reason of intelligence or education; by social, economic or marital status; by religious upbringing, observance or experience. Of course the sort of person who gets ill, his intelligence and background will affect how he deals with his illness, and the sort of family he belongs to will affect how soon and to what extent he realises that he is ill. But none of these things can prevent him from becoming ill.

There is much misunderstanding amongst medical as well as lay people about what psychiatric treatment can hope to achieve. It cannot provide what nature herself has omitted to endow an individual with. It cannot make a short person grow taller, it cannot turn a dull-witted person into a scholar, and it cannot make a naturally retiring bookworm into a gregarious athlete. It can neither give nor take away spiritual life, but it can remove some of the psychological barriers that prevent a person from entering fully into that realm of life.

One aspect of treatment which puzzles and even horrifies people is that it is not unusual for a strong attachment to develop between the patient and his doctor. This marked dependence on and faith in another person is considered by some to be utterly unworthy of a Christian. In fact it is a valuable therapeutic tool. Only when a person has a strong positive relationship of trust can he feel confident enough to reveal his inner world.

This dependence is especially marked in certain forms of treatment that set out to explore emotional difficulties in detail. During the course of it the unconscious conflicts that have caused the disturbance will become evident in the patient's dealings with his doctor. This occurs because there is a tendency to transfer to the doctor, in the present relationship, attitudes that arose from his relationship with other people in the past. In this way his difficulties become more directly open to examination, understanding and eventual correction because they are being experienced at the time when they are under discussion.

As treatment proceeds, the relationship between patient and doctor is likely to go through many different phases. Whatever the phase, the doctor aims to help the patient resolve his own difficulties in a more constructive and mature way.

People who have learnt to regard any expression of anger as bad, or all sexual impulses and feelings as dangerous, have been defrauded. They have been prevented from using two most important sources of energy. The emotion of anger and the arousal of sexual feelings are both essentially creative,

117

God-given energies. A considerable amount of treatment time has to be spent helping some people discover and re-claim these instinctual energies so that they can become the positive, constructive forces that they were intended to be.

Another feature of psychiatric treatment that causes concern is the fear that it will undermine or destroy a person's faith. This cannot happen when that faith is well grounded, but it can (and should) when he uses his religion primarily as an emotional crutch. Those who avoid psychiatric help when it is needed, for fear that they will then lose their faith, would do well to examine on what their faith is based. It may be a house built on shifting sand, not solid rock.

Yet another objection to seeking treatment is the notion that if Christ is supreme then faith in Him should by itself deliver a believer from mental turmoil. That Christ can heal today as completely and instantly as He did when on earth is not doubted, but it would be a miracle and miracles are rare. They are a 'special intervention of God for a religious end, transcend-ing the normal order of things'.[1] Unless there is some good reason for a special intervention, restoration of health will usually be achieved by the normal methods current at the time.

The daily life of Christ gives the greatest example of the economic and purposeful use of miracles. He regularly used a boat when it was necessary to cross the lake, although

[1] *Oxford Dictionary of the Christian Church.*

we know that He could, and sometimes did, walk across on the water when there was a special reason to do so. He can still suspend and reverse natural laws but this is not something which we have any right to expect. Unless there is a special reason for a miracle the natural order of events, and the currently available methods of healing, are not short-circuited.

The fellowship of an active, caring church has a vital contribution to make. Remember the paralysed man who could not get himself to Christ! His friends not only carried him there, but literally tore the roof apart to get him in beside the Lord. It is the responsibility of more fortunate members to help those who are emotionally crippled, for while their emotional problems remain many cannot get themselves to the feet of Jesus. All members of the church have the privilege and the duty to take them there in prayer, and to continue to pray for them until they are able to 'walk' again by themselves.

One can only pray in the most general way for any particular individual during an open prayer meeting. Those with a special knowledge of the needs and difficulties of another will therefore often find it of value to meet together at some other time. Small groups of this nature, meeting on behalf of one or two for whom they have a special concern, can be more specific and detailed in their intercession. Provided that everything that is mentioned really remains confidential this is always to be encouraged.

Great care must, however, be taken to ensure that any talk

about the people prayed for is always absolutely true and absolutely necessary. A prayer gathering must never become a time for speculation or that destructive pastime of gossip.

Imaginative, informed prayer for those in need achieves at least three things. It helps those on whose behalf intercession is made. It influences the attitude of those who pray, making them more understanding and open to the prompting of the Holy Spirit. Also it is often while still at prayer that something which needs doing, and is within the power of the individual to do, comes to mind. When prayer is ended this thought must be translated into action at the appropriate time.

There is much that the Christian Church can, and should, do to bridge the gap between the sick and disturbed person and his neighbour. It has done much for the physically handicapped and for socially deprived children but it has largely ignored the problem of mental illness. For too long the Church has been content to allow mentally disturbed people to be shut away in vast, impersonal, isolated institutions, and with few exceptions it has then proceeded to forget them completely.

Each local church should be actively engaged alongside the professional in this field. It must be alongside and not instead of the professional, because both have their distinctive contribution to make. Christians must bring back the personal touch of concern for the *individual*. Christ calls His own sheep *by name*, yet in every mental hospital there are unnumbered people with no one outside its walls to do this for them, no one to care what happens to them, no one who remembers them.

Many people receive no visits or letters and have no outings year after year. In some the acute illness subsided long ago but after years in a protected environment, totally lacking in stimulation from outside, they remain passive as life passes by. With no one to care about them they have ceased to care about themselves.

Psychiatric illness affects people in various ways, the most universal being that the sufferer feels 'different' and isolated from other people. The essential thing, therefore, is to help him break through his isolation and improve his capacity for healthy personal relationships. It is important to help him keep alive whatever interests he has and to introduce him to new ones whenever possible. He must be helped and encouraged to keep in touch with church and community activities, and this is best done by maintaining personal contact.

People who have had a psychiatric illness often benefit from unobtrusive assistance during their recovery. They need a gradual re-introduction to normal living and are often helped by being invited out for an afternoon, or to spend the day with a family. If they are diffident about returning to a church or social function after an absence, then call for them; make them feel wanted and welcome.

The Church must be above all a caring community. It must accept people as Christ Himself accepts them, which is *just as they happen to be*. However unorthodox, however eccentric and however much they disturb our often rather rigid conception of what people ought to be capable of doing, or of refraining from doing, we are told to 'show no partiality' and to make no distinction in our welcome.

A disturbed person may deviate from the normally accepted pattern of behaviour in a number of ways but his basic need will always be the same. More than anyone else he needs sustained, loving acceptance of himself, even if disapproval has to be expressed about his deviant behaviour. We must, by the grace of God, guard against allowing dislike of a particular method of expressing inner turmoil from turning into dislike and rejection of the disturbed person.

He needs to be loved and accepted for what he actually is, not for what he ought to be, nor for what he might have been. There may have to be a long period of repeatedly finding himself accepted by, and of value to, other people before he can come to accept himself as a member of any community with its reciprocal responsibilities.

In his book *Come Out the Wilderness*[1] Bruce Kenrick gives many examples of this kind of practical Christianity. He tells of how 'this patient, time-consuming visiting, this "wasting time" with people, often made strong human friendships through which lives slowly changed'. He says of one particular parishioner, 'In this way a fragmented existence began to turn into a life.'

A word of caution is necessary here. This is very specialised work—specialised in the human qualities it calls for, the

[1] Published by Fontana.

patience and persistence it requires, and the conviction it demands. Not many people are equipped for it. The average church member must beware of taking on something he cannot continue with. He must consider the possible disruptive effect on his own family and the emotional demands on himself. Most people find it wise to set certain limits to the demands they will meet, in the light of their own circumstances.

Many of the lesser psychological troubles which so many people suffer from today arise from, and are exacerbated by, the isolation and loneliness which have become such a feature of our society. It is increasingly common for people to move away from their families and friends in search of training and employment, and this migration leads to a great deal of bravely hidden loneliness. This needs only a little imagination to detect and relieve.

Strangers should be made welcome not only in the church they attend but also in the homes of its members. Responsibility does not end with a quick recital of mid-week activities and a vague invitation to 'come along any time'. Be definite. Invite the person to come along *with you*, and make a point of introducing him to others. When the newcomer is no longer of an age to be dealt with by an invitation to one of the youth activities, he is more than ever likely to be overlooked if members are intent only on greeting their own particular friends after a service.

To say, 'Do come round one day,' or 'Drop in for coffee any time,' is not enough. Many people are too reserved to take you up on this without more encouragement, so follow it up with a definite, warm invitation. Give a specific time and date, and make it quite clear whether or not a meal is included in the invitation. Some thought is required here. To ask someone round at a time that will mean missing the set meal at their hostel or lodgings is likely to mean an uncomfortable evening, for the guest at least.

If conversation with your guest is hard going, it probably means he needs your companionship and help all the more. Remember this and don't drop him after just one visit, to sink back into loneliness and isolation once again. Search until you find some interest in common that you can share together. Invite other friends round to share the evening. By doing this the task of entertainment is made easier and you give your guest the opportunity of making more acquaintances, some of which may ripen into friendship.

One young church member, on 'look out' duty after the evening service, was amazed to hear that her companion had taken a visitor to the church home to coffee the week before. 'Goodness, I wouldn't like to take a stranger *home*,' she said in horrified tones. Her parents thought that their home was 'open' to all comers; they did not realise that one had to be 'in' before getting there!

Of course there is always the other side to every coin. A woman, well qualified in her profession but constricted in her personality, complained that she could not make friends. In particular she said that no one spoke to her at the church she had recently been attending. She was surprised and at first mystified to be asked how soon after the service she reached home again. She paused before answering, and then became embarrassed. A little honest reflection had quickly shown that she was one of the first out of church. Because of her shyness she did not linger outside but was away down the road before anyone had a chance to talk to her. She thought that the church people were unfriendly and she had not realised what part she herself was playing in her own isolation. It was true that no one spoke to her, but this was more because she denied them the opportunity than because they did not want to be friendly.

An emotionally immature or disturbed person only learns to trust other people when he finds them to be worthy of his trust. A word said lightly, then forgotten; a promise or confidence broken—these things can so easily shatter the trust of someone who is just learning to believe in the good intentions of other people. To help those whose personalities are bruised and damaged is a challenge. We need to go out of our way to meet them, as they are and where they are. Too often we expect them to come to us.

Human resources alone are not sufficient for such a task. Only the love of God, *if allowed to flow through us*, can ever meet such a need. It requires the love that is patient, kind and enduring; the love that is not put off by frequent rebuff; the love that continues to hope for better things and to believe that they will come. The New English Bible rendering of the famous passage in I Corinthians, chapter thirteen puts it like this:

'Love is patient; love is kind and envies no one. Love is

never boastful, nor conceited, nor rude; never selfish, not quick to take offence. Love keeps no score of wrongs; does not gloat over other men's sins, but delights in the truth. There is nothing love cannot face; there is no limit to its faith, its hope, and its endurance.'